Powerlifting Over 50:
Mastering THE Skills for Strength, Health and Vitality

By

Richard Schuller

www.MidLifeHardBody.com

Disclaimer

You should recognize that any exercise program involves some element of risk. You should consult with your physician or health care professional to see if this program is something you can do without endangering your health, and for diagnosis and treatment of illness, injuries and for advice regarding medications.

While exercise is normally beneficial, it is important that you undertake knowing that you do not have any health conditions that may be aggravated or damaged by activities in this program. The author and Mid Life Hard Body, LLC shall have neither liability nor responsibility to any person or entity with respect to any damage or injury alleged to be caused directly or indirectly by the information contained in this book.

You should never discontinue taking medications prescribed by your doctor without specific consultation with your doctor. You should obtain clearance from your doctor before you undertake any program of exercise as the activities may be too strenuous or dangerous for some people.

Before making any changes to your personal diet and nutrition habits it is recommended that you consult with your physician or health care professional. The nutrition information and suggestions in this book are for informational purposes only. While every attempt has been made to verify the accuracy of information provided in all portions of this book, neither the author, nor any affiliate s/partners assume any responsibility for errors, inaccuracies or omissions.

The information contained in this book is not intended for the treatment or prevention of disease, nor as a substitute for medical treatment. The nutrition information in this book should not be adopted without consultation with a physician or your health care professional. Use of information contained in any portion of this book is the sole responsibility of the reader. Neither the author nor any affiliate s/partner is responsible or liable for any harm or injury resulting from the exercises, nutrition advice, or personal management strategies.

www.MidLifeHardBody.com

Copyright 2016 by Richard Schuller

No part of this book may be copied, reproduced, or transmitted without express written permission of the author. This includes any means of sharing, including photocopying, recording, or through any electronic or mechanical means. The only exceptions are portions of the text used in critical reviews or by other means allowed by copyright laws. All rights are reserved.

www.MidLifeHardBody.com

Your purchase does not grant you any authorization to reproduce this product or portions thereof. All rights are reserved by the author, including any distribution or reproduction of the product.

Acknowledgements

As I built this book from the first concept to the final words on the page, I got help and support from some very special people.

My wonderful wife Susan helped make the writing immeasurably better. Her gifts as a screenwriter helped me in more ways than I can count. She helped me clarify the most important information to include in the text. She was a skilled reviewer and editor, and she has also been a constant source of inspiration.

I want to sincerely thank Scott Tousignant who kept encouraging me throughout the writing. He was a perceptive sounding board for many of the ideas included in here. He has been my mentor and friend for several years. His help and guidance have been critical for me.

Special Thanks

To Adam Neiffer and the men and women at Cross Fit Fort Vancouver, thanks for all the help in producing this book. Several members eagerly posed for demonstration photographs. Owner Adam Neiffer generously gave me access to the building and equipment on multiple occasions.

After training in different gyms for nearly 60 years I can honestly say that in my opinion CrossFit Fort Vancouver is one of the best gyms on the planet. The positive energy and genuine friendliness (not to mention curiosity) of everyone makes it an ideal place to train.

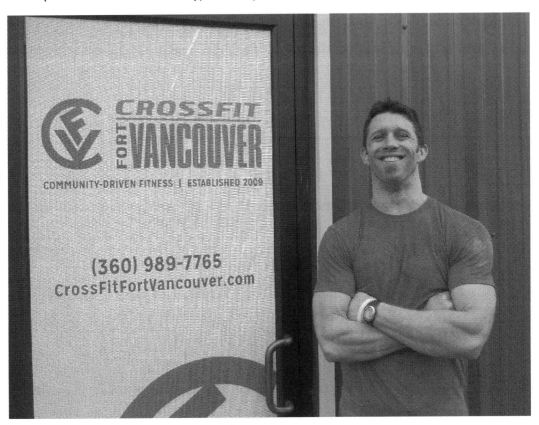

While Cross Fit is more often associated with Olympic style competitive lifting, I found that the staff and members of CF Fort Vancouver eagerly embraced many insights from powerlifting. We have enjoyed a rich exchange of ideas on training, conditioning and life.

Again, my sincere thanks for all your support and assistance in producing this book.

Table of Contents

Introduction

Part I – The Big Picture: Powerlifting and Fitness — 9
Chapter 1 – Powerlifting training over age 50 — 10
Chapter 2 - Developing powerlifting unique athletic skills — 17
Chapter 3- Sport specific conditioning: an overlooked factor — 32
Chapter 4- Training for power: Building training plans — 48

Part II – Training Programs — 62
Chapter 5- The Squat: King of power exercises – proper technique — 65
Chapter 6- Training cycles for the squat — 86
    Cycle 1: Foundation cycle — 90
    Cycle 2: Partial squats and deep pauses — 95
    Cycle 3: Elastic Band Training — 100
    Cycle 4: Box squats and front squats — 107
    Cycle 5: Peaking program — 115
Chapter 7- Bench Press: THE most popular lift – proper technique — 122
Chapter 8- Bench Press training cycles — 142
    Cycle 1: Foundation cycle — 143
    Cycle 2: Explosive strength I — 147
    Cycle 3: Power cage training — 151
    Cycle 4: Explosive strength II — 157
    Cycle 5: Peaking program — 162
Chapter 9 – Deadlift: Pulling monster iron -technique and core assistance — 173
Chapter 10 – Deadlift training cycles — 195
    Cycle 1: Foundation cycle — 196
    Cycle 2: Strength builder cycle — 199
    Cycle 3: Elastic band training — 203
    Cycle 4: Power max cycle — 209
    Cycle 5: Peaking cycle — 211
Chapter 11 – Isometrics: A forgotten training method that promotes big gains — 218

Part III – Getting the most from your training — 232
Chapter 12 – Pathway to success: small steps to big improvements — 233
Chapter 13 – Nutrition for power — 251
Chapter 14 – Overtraining and injuries — 260
Chapter 15- Supplements and performance enhancing drugs: A cautionary tale — 266
Chapter 16- Entering a powerlifting meet: a step by step guide — 274

Afterword — 296

Introduction

Powerlifting Over 50: A *great* way to be *both* fit and strong.

Powerlifting is one of the greatest activities you can do that can give you both serious fitness and phenomenal strength. You can also look great, have a ton of personal confidence and enjoy your workouts like never before.

You don't *have* to compete, you just train like you *were going to compete.* You get the benefits either way.

Training for powerlifting has a lot of perks for people over 50 in addition to looking years younger and having the actual body of someone *much* younger.

The cool thing about the sport of powerlifting is that you can do it at a very high level for an incredibly long time. I should know. I spent 25 years competing and "retired" at the tender age of 72. I could still do it, but a quarter century of lifting at a national and international level seemed like "enough". I was ready for a new challenge.

I can say without the slightest reservation that I loved powerlifting, loved competing and above all loved "lifting heavy stuff". I know a lot of people who love to "lift heavy stuff" who might never want to compete. Still, they want to lift as much as they can.

This book is for all the people who like lifting heavy stuff, who want to maximize what they can lift. It is structured around training for competition, but training that way, in my opinion, is the best way to get in really great condition.

I like to think of this book as being aimed at the "lions and tigers" over the age of 50. There are some ways that you have to train a little differently than kids in their 20's, but you can still produce monster lifts. You just have to be a little more careful and deliberate about it than someone with only two or three decades of life experience.

I thought you might want to know something about me, since I'll be offering you a lot of advice in the coming pages.

I have based this book on my 25 years as a competing lifter, the coaching I got from some of the greats in the sport, and constant research I did during my lifting career. I was also a national referee for 20+ years, and got to see a vast number of mistakes that lifters made on the platform. I learned a LOT from this experience.

During my lifting career, my professional life was as a research scientist in a private R & D firm. My work life could not have been more different than my sporting background. However, I used my skills as a researcher to dig into advanced training methods, new (or ancient) ideas about physical fitness and strength, and searching for approaches that would enable me to excel at the sport I loved.

www.MidLifeHardBody.com

My experience with weight lifting began in (gasp!) 1955. I was a relatively fast, but very spindly 14-year-old who wanted to play high school football...without getting killed. I was an imposing physical specimen of 5'9" and 130 pounds. This was two decades before football players lifted weights, and there were no barbells in our high school.

In the spring of 1955, I found some bodybuilding magazines in the local drug store. It was immediately evident that additional muscle on me could make a big difference in my life expectancy on the football field. So, I sent off an order to Joe Weiders factory in New Jersey, and was rewarded with 300 pounds of "freight" arriving at the Railway Express office on the last day of school my freshman year.

Over the summer I followed the Weider beginners course lifting three times a week, ate a lot, and worked at a summer job. I didn't notice that my shirts were getting really tight, nor did I step on the scale. However, when I reported for football practice in mid-August I had added 30 pounds of muscle. The coaches were (pleasantly) shocked. As I said, at that time, no one who played sports lifted weights.

I continued to lift all through high school, and added wrestling to my list of sports. When I graduated, I was still the only player on my team (and probably the only player in the conference) who lifted weights.

When I started college at Michigan State in the fall of 1958, I quickly found the weight room where one of the legends of Olympic style lifting, Pat O'Shea, presided as coach. I was totally hooked, and competed in Olympic lifting for the three years it took me to graduate.

During this time, I had the great good fortune to meet one of greatest lifters the US ever produced. The legendary Olympic champion Norbert Shemansky showed me what focus and hard work were needed to excel.

After spending just short of four years in the Navy, I headed for graduate school at the University of Oregon. Again, I began training for Olympic style weightlifting, but there were no other competitive lifters, and nowhere to compete. As Oregon was a great track school, I gravitated to the company of the runners, and began what would be a 22-year career in foot racing.

In the early days, I ran sprints. At the time the only races available were longer runs, so I moved to longer distances. This was before the "running boom" and most foot races drew a handful of participants. As in my weightlifting career, I had the great good fortune to learn from some of the best runners in the world at the time.

My first job was as a professor at the University of Tennessee and a scientist at the Oak Ridge National Laboratory. I quickly got involved with the running scene in eastern Tennessee and competed with friends in the Knoxville Track Club for the five years I spent there.

www.MidLifeHardBody.com

As I said before, all this happened before what would be called the "running boom". Foot races drew a handful of participants. For example, the famed Atlanta Peachtree Run drew about 160 of us the first year it was held. I think that now it draws 20-30,000.

In 1975 I moved from Knoxville, TN to a new job in Seattle, WA. This was a hotbed of running and for the next 12 years, I competed in foot racing at every distance from 100 meters to 15 miles. And then...I got really bored with running.

My weightlifting career was reignited when I joined a new gym in Issaquah, WA.

Powerliting had not existed as a sport when I had previously competed in weightlifting. However, I immediately embraced the "new to me" sport of powerlifting. Heavy squats, bench press and deadlift offered formidable and rewarding challenges. I started with local meets, and by 1990 had qualified for the drug free national masters' championships.

What may be interesting to those of you who are over 50 is that I *began* my powerlifting career at age 47 and started competing nationally at age 50. You see, it is never too late to...get started.

Not being content with lifting alone, I became a certified national referee in 1990 and officiated at more meets than I can remember for the next 22 years.

For a ten-year stretch in the 2000's I became a meet promoter. I put on meets with my business partner and friend, Andrew "Bull" Stewart. Together we put on 3 lifting meets a year for a decade. Our state championship meet became one of the largest powerlifting meets in the United States.

After 25 years in the sport, I did my last competitive meet in December 2012. I had no regrets about "retiring" from a 25-year career in a sport that I loved. I had a great time, made a lot of friends, and reached a venerable age with great physical health and strength.

Did I quit and "go to seed"? No way...being fit and strong is waaaay too much fun....

But....this book was written so that *you* could set personal records, improve your "game" and enjoy the sport. Go for it!

Richard Schuller

Portland, OR

March 2016

www.MidLifeHardBody.com

Part I

The Big Picture:
Powerlifting and Fitness

Food for Thought:

"If you live hard, life is easy; if you live easy, live is *hard!*"
Dan John

"The less a person knows about something, the less they think there is to know...."
David McRaney

"Give me patience, and I want it NOW!"
-anonymous

Chapter 1

Powerlifting Training Over age 50

Why do we love powerlifting so much? Everyone has their own personal reasons, but at least one of them is that powerlifting is a *real* competitive sport for anyone over 50 (or any age) because it is done in age groups. You compete against people your own age.

Other reasons we love the sport is that it can be exhilarating, rewarding, fun, exciting, and can give you a deep sense of personal satisfaction. (It can also be frustrating, but that seems to pass quickly).

Of course another big benefit is that you can get into *extraordinary* physical condition.

If you are over 50, you can have a *great experience* doing powerlifting. This book is designed to help *you* get all the fun, satisfaction and joy that you can from this difficult and demanding sport. In short, the information that follows is designed to help *you* be the best you can be.

How long can you continue to lift heavy and get the benefits of this uniquely special activity?

Powerlifting is one of the sports that you can compete in almost indefinitely. I should know. I had a 25-year career as a powerlifter that *began* when I was 48. That means I did my last competitive meet at age 72. Now at age 75, I don't compete, but still lift serious iron. I'm in near bulletproof shape and I know that with about three months of preparation, I could easily compete again.

While a lot of my age peers have problems getting out of a chair, it is really a kick to contemplate doing heavy squats...or pulling deadlifts that would cripple some people.

Most people who exercise want to look good. Almost everyone who does powerlifting training develops a very *athletic* looking body. Most powerlifters develop a lean muscular look that is universally appealing. You don't get huge and freaky looking unless you overeat and take a bunch of banned drugs. I can tell you it is amazing to still have this athletic look at 75.

Another aspect of powerlifting that is very appealing to many people is that you measure your progress *objectively*. Weights you lift weigh exactly what they weigh. There is lift, there is no fuzzy, arbitrary, subjective

I wrote this book for two groups of people: those who want to compete in the sport, and those who don't want to compete but want to use powerlifting training to get into great physical condition. The same program works for both.

Whatever your goal, it is my hope that you can have as much fun as I did...and be the very best lifter you can be.

This book is designed to help you get the most out of your training, and put up the biggest lifts your body can perform. To achieve this after age 50, you will need to use the most powerful "muscle" in your body...your mind. You are going to have to maximize your ability to plan, isolate training problems, and execute your strategies by *thinking carefully* about them.

Powerlifting: Part of a Proud Tradition

Performing feats of genuine strength has been a respected part of civilized cultures for thousands of years. From the earliest Greek athletes to the current day weightlifters, the ability to do authentic feats of strength has been respected in every advanced culture.

Powerlifting is part of an ancient tradition of strong men and now women. When you take up powerlifting, you become part of this tradition. Thousands before you have performed the feats of strength that were the most respected in their day. You have chosen to take on the strength challenges of the present day.

Feats of strength are respected because they are very hard to accomplish. Things that are easily done are commonplace.

People marvel at feats of strength because they are *real*. There is no trickery or illusion about them. Success in strength comes only from hard work, determination, refusal to be defeated, relentless practice, and constant working to improve. Success cannot be purchased or faked.

There is no concealing success or failure. Powerlifting is done with the lifter alone on a platform with three judges determining compliance with the rules, and an audience who sees everything. There is no place to hide. There is no way to lie about the outcome. Lifting is done in the open for everyone to see. Talk means nothing.

When a lifter goes on the platform, the weight to be lifted is the same whether the lifter is a billionaire or a humble high school student. There is no allowance for social status, political connections, ethnicity, or nation of birth. One hundred kilograms is one hundred kilograms for everyone.

Powerlifting is not for the meek. It is extremely difficult to do, and requires that you push yourself in ways you may never have thought possible. A famous quote from Theodore Roosevelt sums this up:

It is not the critic who counts; not the man who points out how the strong man stumbles, or where the doer of deeds could have done them better. The credit belongs to the man who is actually in the arena, whose face is marred by dust and sweat and blood; who strives valiantly; who errs, who comes short again and again, because there is no effort without error and shortcoming; but who does actually strive to do the deeds; who knows great enthusiasms, the great devotions; who spends himself in a worthy cause; who at the best knows in the end the triumph of high achievement, and who at the worst, if he fails, at least fails while daring greatly, so that his place shall never be with those cold and timid souls who neither know victory nor defeat.

You are part of a tradition that is old, respected and hard. Respect the sport, and be joyful in the precious opportunity you have to carry on the tradition.

Powerlifting Over 50: What's Different?

In contrast to the usual cliché's about "inevitable decline", the news for powerlifters over 50 is really great. If you are among the senior contingent, there is indisputable evidence that you can become *insanely* strong. You can do big lifts that will stun people 30 years younger.

There really are far fewer limits on your potential than is commonly believed.

How can you realize your full potential?

The key will be to make use of your biggest assets, life experience and your (by now) well developed intelligence to train "smart". This is not to say you won't train hard, but it emphasizes that you will use your smarts, common sense and ability to learn to craft a maximally effective program to become seriously strong.

What is different after age 50?

Two things:

- Things you do better than younger lifters
- Things that require additional attention and care

What do you do better than younger lifters?

The main things in this category are the ability to use your mind, and your life experience to know your body better, train smarter and learn new skills.

As I will say over and over again, *strength is a skill*. It can be very hard for younger lifters to have the patience to master a difficult skill. Being a superior lifter is about mastering skills. My observations lead me to believe that a lot of young athletes want instant gratification

Older lifters will take the time and have the patience to really nail the skill aspects of powerlifting.

Better skill yields better performance. Better skill means you can get much closer to your biological limit than someone who is trying to lift on emotion and adrenalin.

Experienced athletes are usually able to compete more effectively, because the "pressure" of competition does not get to them the way it does to less experienced lifters. This can take the form of anything from reacting to missing a lift, to training or competing in unfamiliar places, to dealing with any difficult circumstance. Much more on this later.

Finally, if you have been training steadily for a long time, you will have built up an unbelievable amount of basic body strength. Body strength declines very slowly as we age, and if you have been training for a long time, your baseload body strength will stay with you for what seems like forever.

Younger lifters don't have the accumulated body strength that comes from years of training. Thus they are somewhat less resilient when it comes to recovering from heavy training. Younger lifters may also not have toughened tendons and ligaments that come from long years moving big iron.

Finally, the biggest advantage older lifters have is that they *can* have the sense to "train smart" rather than simply blast away and train as hard as they can. The old lions may not put in all the gym reps that the cub does, but the older folks will get more out of what they do.

Areas where attention and care are important

One of the biggest problems older lifters face: recovering from heavy training.

In general, older lifters recover more slowly than they did in their younger years. "Training smart", you will take this into account, and not over train. Your progress in lifting will be limited by your recovery….so pay as much attention to recovering as you would to any other critical factor in your training.

If you have been lifting weights for years, I want to explain that lifting *heavy weights* is NOT the same activity as lifting lighter weights. Lifting heavy requires a unique type of muscular conditioning and endurance that is different from that needed for training with light weights. You will have a head start on someone who has not been lifting before, but be aware that you need to work into heavy lifting gradually.

If you have NOT been training for some time, even a few months, it is critical that you get back into heavy lifting slowly. If you try to do too much weight or too much of a workload before your body is ready for it, you are at risk for a significant injury. This will set you back months, or even longer.

If you have been in training and/or sports for many years, you will probably have some cumulative wear and tear on your joints and connective tissue. If you are still in the game, you probably have learned how to keep these injuries at bay so you can keep playing hard.

Remember, the sports doctors and the physical therapists are your pals. They can be huge in helping you have a great lifting career. Don't hesitate to learn about the good ones who practice close to where you live.

Bottom line: older people recover from heavy training more slowly than younger ones. But, if you manage your recovery and condition yourself to lift heavy, you can get great results.

Then there is metabolism: it declines slowly as you age, so you will probably need to eat less than you did when you were 30, or even 40. Extra chow tends to quickly become "table muscle" (aka. "fat"), and you don't want extra portions of that stuff hanging around you.

Each person has unique dietary needs. You will probably need to spend some time figuring out what pattern of eating is best for you. For example, I tend to eat one main meal a day, have some small snacks, and have a 14-16-hour period when I eat nothing. This works great for me. However, my wife found that this pattern made her feel awful. She now has a completely different pattern from me.

You may find is that you need more sleep than you did in your 30's. Extra sleep is one of the few "silver bullets" for better strength and health. You will see a lot of references to the huge power of sleep throughout this book.

Finally, like it or not, it may take longer to recover from injury than it did when you were younger. Obviously, do all you can to avoid getting injured. If you do get hurt, be diligent about your recovery, and you will be back training again. This will never happen as fast as you want it to, but you can shorten the time by "training smart.

Becoming a better powerlifter

It really helps if you understand the "big picture" of what you are trying to do. A good place to start is breaking down how you think about your task of becoming a better lifter.

If you ask the average lifter if they would like to make significant improvements on their strength, everyone will quickly say "yes". It is easy to "want" to be stronger, but doing what is necessary to get there is far more of a challenge.

In this book I'll give you a guide on how to improve your lifting. The approach may be different from what you are used to seeing. I break down the process of making improvements into the following areas:

- Improving the *sport specific skills* needed to improve
- Doing the *sport specific conditioning* needed to train hard
- Understanding the *pathway to success:* desire, persistence and planning
- *Doing the work*, and monitoring your progress

All of these elements systematically fit together to help you to become the best lifter you can be. Let's look at each one.

Sport Specific Skills

Every sport has some unique skills that must be learned in order to participate, and *mastered* in order to excel. It doesn't matter what the sport may be, there are certain specific skills that form the core of what you do.

For example, in baseball one must learn to hit the ball with a bat, play the field, throw, catch, etc. In tennis it is necessary to learn how to hit the ball with a racquet, and then make the ball go where you want it to go. In basketball, you have to learn how to handle the ball, shoot and play the floor.

Each sport has its unique skill set. It is the same in powerlifting.

However, many lifters tend to overlook this critical fact. Too often the specific skill part of power training is either unrecognized or ignored. In this book I will devote a lot of attention to the athletic skills specific to lifting big iron.

Sport Specific Conditioning

People who train with weights will "lift weights". However, the conditioning needed for Olympic Style weightlifting, bodybuilding and powerlifting is drastically different.

Again, this seems obvious, but too often I have found that powerlifters ignore their own unique conditioning requirements, and suffer poor performance or significant injury as a consequence.

Later, I'll lay out some sport specific conditioning exercises that should be part of every powerlifters workout.

Pathway to Success

As all of you know, no one achieves anything serious by accident. There are a sequence of things that must happen for someone to go from novice to expert. I have attempted to set these out in a logical manner so that they are easy to follow.

In simple words, the pathway to success begins with a desire to achieve something. Without this nothing more will happen.

This desire must be coupled with a fierce persistence, or all activity will stop at the first sign of difficulty.

Finally, the energy and determination must be focused through a plan for getting from where one is now to where one wants to go. No plan, no success.

Do the work!

It is critical to make plans as they are the roadmap to success. However, plans without execution are useless.

Real progress comes from doing the work defined in the plans. This requires a clear intention to do what is needed, and then the allocation of time and effort necessary.

A critical element in making progress is a system for monitoring what is being done, and how well it is working. The "feedback" function is essential if one wants to know if what they are doing is actually achieving what they want.

Format of the Book

In Part I of the book I'll give you the "Big Picture". This is an overview of factors that are critical to your success as a lifter. There is a lot of information you won't see anywhere else, and this section is aimed at helping you structure all your training to produce maximum gains.

I'll introduce some ideas that may be totally new to you, but in my view are absolutely critical to realizing your full potential as a lifter. These include sport specific skills and sport specific conditioning.

I'll go into detail about how you plan and execute your training. This is vital because so few lifters actually maximize their returns from planning their training, focusing on continuing improvement, and using feedback to obtain continuing progress.

A lot of Part I will be focused on the unique athletic skills you need to develop to excel, the type of conditioning you need for heavy lifting, and then how to construct a training plan that will get you where you want to go.

In Part II, I'll present specific training routines for the Squat, Bench Press and Deadlift. By using the planning methods described in Part I, you will be able to structure your own training programs.

In Part III, I cover the critical mental aspects of doing your best and things in your head that might subvert your progress, supplements, risks of performance enhancing drugs, and a step by step guide to entering and competing in a powerlifting meet.

The intention is that you be able to use this as a reference guide throughout many years of training. If you follow the routines in this book, you will be able to make major progress in building your strength for as long as you want to lift.

Enjoy the journey.

Chapter 2

Developing Powerlifting Unique Athletic Skills

Powerlifting unique athletic skills

Let me introduce the area of powerlifting unique athletic skills by stating one poorly understood fact:

Lifting heavy weights is a very different activity than lifting light weights.

It may appear that one goes through some of the same motions lifting both light and heavy weights, but the ability to lift heavy is very different than lifting light.

What is different?

First of all, lifting light weights does not require that you activate the muscle fibers to their full capacity. When you lift heavy, the idea is to mobilize 100% of your muscle fibers in a maximum lift. Typical gym lifting may only require that the muscle work at 60-80% of maximum.

A second very critical difference is the when lifting light weights, little demand is placed on the coordinated application of force by several different muscle groups. Light weights don't place demands on stabilizer muscle groups, or require the quick transfer of heavy loads from one set of muscles to another.

Third, heavy lifting requires the ability to maximally contract certain muscles, while relaxing others to allow for a coordinated movement of the weight. For example, descending in a heavy squat requires that your glutes and hamstrings be somewhat relaxed. When you begin to drive upward out of the bottom, the glutes and hamstrings have to be contracted with maximum force.

Fourth, lifting heavy weights require that you control the weight in space while the weight is moving. This requires that virtually every muscle in your body work in a coordinated manner. With a light weight, controlling the weight in space requires little or no intermuscular coordination.

As long as you train with weights, remember the fundamental fact:

Strength is a Skill and Skills can be Learned!

The *skill* in powerlifting is to mobilize maximum force into each competitive lift.

This was first brought to my attention by the great Pavel Tsatsouline. This seemingly simple phrase has huge implications for everything you must do to improve your powerlifting.

Few lifters have any idea of how to mobilize maximum force for heavy lifting. This is because most either train for other purposes, or have never been taught how to put out max power.

One of the big problems in learning how to mobilize maximum force is that it is *very difficult to observe* this particular lifting skill. Let me give you an example.

Think about a sport like platform diving where, like powerlifting, you complete the competition activity in a few seconds. It is obvious even to the casual observer that doing a great dive from the 10-meter board requires a lot of highly developed skill.

In powerlifting the skills needed for great performance are virtually impossible to observe directly, because they all take place *inside the body*. But, to lift heavy weights, it is absolutely necessary to develop the skills that will enable you to do what is needed to move big iron.

Powerlifting is unlike diving in that the casual observer cannot "see" the difference between a great lift and a crappy one. To the average person, and the average lifter, both the great squat and the garbage version look like pretty much the same movement.

Nothing could be further from the truth.

I believe that because it is so hard to "see" how much skill is involved in lifting heavy weights, many lifters are unaware of how critical these skill sets are to maximum performance. Thus, they don't train to develop and perfect these skills and their lifting totals suffer as a result.

Realizing your full potential as a lifter will mean *developing the skill*s needed for heavy lifting. This involves mastering many physical skills that are completely "inside" the body, and are hard to observe from the outside.

Here are the unique athletic skills that are necessary in *all* of the power lifts:

- Balance and intermuscular coordination
- *Recruiting* every muscle in the body to provide power for the lift
- Getting "tight" and staying tight during the lift
- Ability to put out 100% effort into a 1 repetition maximum lift
- Perfect form to obtain maximum mechanical advantage and do a competition legal lift

Developing a Skill

Most of us have heard the old saying that "practice makes perfect". That is true *only if you practice the right things and practice them correctly.*

When you begin the quest to build or enhance a skill set, I believe it is important to understand some important characteristics of "skill".

Initially, think of skills in an area in terms of *levels* of ability. In simple terms, there are low, medium and high levels of skill in *all areas of activity*. For example, think of three different skill sets: riding a bike, playing the piano and powerlifting.

Thinking of the three different skill sets, at low levels of skill, a person could ride a bike, play simple tunes, and lift a few weights. At a mid-level of skill, a person could do trail riding, play a few songs, and workout with weights regularly.

People with high levels of skills in these three areas could be: competing in bike racing, performing piano professionally, or competing in powerlifting.

Reaching the low level of ability in any one of these areas is not very demanding. Obviously it takes some persistence to practice a few elementary skills until one can ride a bike without training wheels, play chopsticks, and do basic weight lifting movements.

Reaching the mid-level of skill takes more persistence and practice. But, becoming modestly skilled means becoming proficient at the *elementary* skill set. That means that the main thing needed to achieve mid-level competence in most things is to repeatedly practice the simplest elements of the skill set.

Reaching high levels of skill is a more demanding task than acquiring low or medium levels of skill. The skills needed at a high level are much more complex than the simple skills needed to do something at a novice level. The practice mantra now is "do the *right things* and *do them right* or fail to improve".

This simple saying has huge implications for becoming highly skilled as a powerlifter.

In my six decades in sports I have come to the conclusion that most people reach a certain modest level of performance and then never get any better for three reasons:

- They don't know *what* to practice to get better, so they continue to practice what they learned in the elementary stages of training
- They are *satisfied* with their current level of achievement
- They are *frustrated* by the difficulty of learning more demanding skills

If you don't know what to practice, what do you do? Do what you already know how to do. This results in a situation where people diligently practice doing things that are either wrong or completely ineffective.

When it comes to being satisfied with one's current level of skill, there are some different reasons for this. The first would be that without further improvement, you are "good enough".

For example, I am a regular golfer. I play at least twice a decade. I feel my existing level of skill is enough to meet this challenge.

Another reason people will stop trying to improve is that they believe it is too much work to work to *master* a skill.

The point is that to realize one's full potential, it is necessary to practice developing needed skills that are difficult and often elusive. This is certainly true in golf, powerlifting, mathematics, music, and so forth.

Over my six decades in sports I have come to the conclusion that most people use "practice" to perfect their mistakes or quit trying to improve at a point far below their real potential.

Do not fall into the trap of believing that "going through the motions" will get you very far. This is settling for being mediocre.

Your mantra going forward should be "*perfect* *practice makes perfect*". In this book, I'll present skills to *practice and perfect* if you want to be a better powerlifter.

Learning the skills of strength is really like being a good piano player. On piano, once you have reached a high level of skill, you have to continue to practice at a demanding level of precision or you begin to sound less like a pro and more like you are wearing winter gloves when you play.

This is because a lot of high level skills are *perishable*. They will erode if not practiced perfectly on a regular basis.

In powerlifting, you first need to master the sport specific skills needed to excel. Then, you need to keep practicing these skills so that your capabilities are kept at a very high level. If you don't practice strength skills, your lifts will decline, or never improve.

When doing power training, always treat every session as an opportunity to build or enhance your sport specific skills. If you don't a sinister thing may happen. You may actually see some of your skills begin to erode.

You cannot turn the skill on and off any more than a piano player can be sloppy in practice and expect to play well in a concert.

Here are four skills you will have to develop to reach your full potential as a powerlifter.

- Balance and Intermuscular Coordination
- Recruiting muscles
- Getting and staying "tight"
- Ability to put out 100% for a single repetition

Balance, Stability and Intermuscular Coordination

Lifting big weights depends on your ability to control heavy weights in space and put out maximum force while standing on your feet. To control your body in this way requires that you have excellent balance and stability, which allows you to exert maximum force while doing the lift.

Having a stable base requires that a large number of muscles work in a *coordinated* manner to keep the athlete properly aligned during the lift. Stabilizers for heavy lifting include all the muscles in the legs, back, abdomen, shoulders, and neck. In short, all the muscles in the body become involved in lifting big weights at some point during a squat, bench press or deadlift.

When lifting light weights, stability is rarely an issue. When lifting heavy weights, having a stable base is absolutely necessary, or a lot of energy and force is dissipated fighting for balance and control. Thus, the first step in lifting big weights is to have a stable base.

Few people ever pay any attention to developing a completely stable base when doing typical fitness workouts. Training with relatively light weight requires only minimal support muscle activation.

Developing the skill needed to lift heavy weights begins with establishing stability while standing on your feet, and then training the body's stabilizer muscles to work together while moving big iron.

As people age, one of the things that tends to happen is that many stabilizer muscles become dormant because they are unused. Muscles degenerate or become "switched off" by the brain if they are not used for a long period of time. Among the first to go are those that stabilize your body during walking or standing.

Even if you are relatively active, there can be muscle groups that you ignore for a while, and they get lazy. Thus, some basic balance skills have eroded. For example, how many 50 year olds do you know who can stand on one foot for more than a few seconds?

The starting point for building the skill to lift big weights is rock solid balance.

Building balance starts with training your brain to activate the support muscles you need to control heavy weights.

The cool thing about approaching power training with this idea is that regardless of your age, your brain can "learn" to activate muscles in ways that you may not have used for a very long time. Learning to lift big weights is going to involve *training your brain to send new messages to your muscles.* This is a part of what I call *learning the skill of strength.*

There are some basic stabilizer drills that you should routinely practice to build your ability to exert maximum force in a coordinated manner.

The first step is training to be stable and balanced on each of your feet while standing.

Begin your balance training by focusing on using your 2nd and 3rd toes to be the primary stabilizer of your foot. You may notice that as you walk these toes have been relaxed or "uninvolved" in your step. When that happens, you may unconsciously be standing with many of your stabilizer muscles "turned off".

To start getting the stabilizer muscles activated, you should regularly practice standing on one foot. See if you can stand on one foot for 30 seconds. When you have mastered that, begin moving your opposite leg into different positions and try to keep your balance. These drills will help you activate the neural pathways that allow for greater muscular control.

You don't have to do this in a gym, you can do it any time you feel like it. An easy time to practice standing on one foot is between sets during your workout. Over time, you will build your ability to better maintain your balance.

The next thing you should do is to focus on generating stability while standing on two feet. The easiest way to do this is to consciously dig your toes into the floor while you are handling the weight. This activates the stabilizer muscles and will train your body so that eventually activating the stabilizer muscles will be automatic.

Another part of promoting maximum power output while standing is to think of your foot being divided down the middle from the toes to the heel. The inside part (big toe side) is where you generate power. The outside half is for balance. When you pull a deadlift, or push upward on a squat, the inside half of your foot will be where the force is focused.

Here are two drills to help you establish a stable base while squatting. Use a light weight and do full squats while standing on a gym mat. Keeping control of the squat bar on an unstable surface will activate all of your stabilizer muscles.

Next, try squatting while blindfolded. Lack of visual ques will really challenge your ability to do a full squat properly. Your stabilizer muscles will be fully activated.

I suggest you begin by doing both of these drills in a power cage, or with a spotter so you don't risk getting hurt.

You can enhance your deadlift strength with a simple drill. Stand on one foot, bent over at the waist, with you opposite leg out behind you. Hold this position for 10-15 seconds. Stand on one foot with each leg. You will enhance your stability for the pull significantly.

Another exercise that has great stability benefit is one leg deadlifts. Start with a light kettlebell and do several reps with each leg. Regular practice on this lift will help you develop and keep good balance for lifting.

Recruiting muscles

Nearly everyone who has trained with weights has heard about the idea of "isolation". This is the practice of focusing on a specific muscle group, and doing exercises that are designed to build those muscles exclusively. An example would be using the leg extension machine to build the quadriceps.

This training does not involve other muscle groups, and while it will stimulate growth in the quadriceps, the movement will do nothing for the hamstrings, glutes, abdominals, etc. Training on the quad machine will not do anything to enhance the *coordinated* use of different muscle groups. The effect will be on the quads in "isolation".

Isolation is <u>*exactly the opposite*</u> of what you need to do in order to build body power. A powerful body is not merely a "collection of parts", it is a powerful <u>*system.*</u> This means that in heavy lifting, the body works as a complete coordinated unit, not as one muscle group moving the load.

To get a <u>*powerful system*</u> working, it is essential that the lifter <u>*recruit*</u> every muscle group to move the weight.

When I discuss proper lifting technique in later sections, I will always emphasize how proper form can facilitate muscle recruiting. For now, simply be aware that your mantra should be "recruit, recruit, recruit". That is a huge factor in how much you will eventually be able to lift.

When done properly, all three power lifts (squat, bench press and deadlift) are literally "whole body lifts". Every muscle in the body *should* contribute to a max lift. This is as true with the bench press as it is with the squat or deadlift.

The emphasis is on "should". Most people *do not* mobilize all their muscular resources when doing a big lift. Many have learned bad habits from doing what I call "general gym training". That is, doing exercises with no attention to proper technique or muscle mobilization.

Right from the start of your power training, you need to think about *recruiting* all of your muscles to produce maximum power. This involves consciously bringing all of your muscles into a state of tension, and keeping them there during your lifting.

The great Pavel Tsatsouline had a very simple demonstration of the power of muscle recruitment that everyone should try for themselves.

With a strong partner, grasp one of his hands in a handshake. Leave your opposite hand relaxed while you squeeze his hand as hard as you can. Feel the force you generate on his hand. Then, while you continue to squeeze as hard as you can, make a tight fist with the hand that had been relaxed. You will feel a surge of power into your opposite hand...the one in the handshake.

You thought you had been squeezing as hard as you could, but with other muscle groups relaxed, you could not generate maximum force. Bringing *all* your muscles into play increases the force you can generate.

Amplifying force is absolutely critical when you are trying to do heavy power lifts. You *must recruit every ounce of force you can.* This means consciously focusing on involving every muscle into the lifting effort.

Recruiting literally means practicing the "feel" of consciously involving every muscle group in your body into a given lift. For example, when you do the bench press, you should *consciously* tighten your entire body. This includes, back, arms, legs, glutes, abs and calves. No muscle group is left out. When you push the weight off your chest, you should "feel" the push in the balls of your feet, your abs should push against your lifting belt, your glutes should contract, and so forth.

Many trainees develop bad habits over the years of relaxing some part of their body when they do a lift. You have to assess whether you are doing this, and take immediate steps to recruit all the muscles that have been taking time off.

The key to recruiting every muscle group in your body begins with getting your entire body "tight" (and keeping it that way). When all your muscles are tensed, you can begin to train yourself to put out maximum

Getting and staying "tight"

The main way you recruit muscles to contribute to a max lift is by "getting tight". This means that when you prepare to lift a heavy weight, you tighten up your *entire body.* Being tight will allow you to put everything you have into a specific lift.

Learning how to get your body into a state of maximum tension takes a while if you have not done it before. You have to learn how to develop full body tension for the squat, bench press and deadlift.

It is often hard to see lifters getting "tight" because all the muscle action occurs *inside* the body. A lifter who is locked down tight ready to deadlift looks virtually identical to one who is partially or completely relaxed.

So, training on becoming tight is something that has to happen in a way that your "feel" when muscles are locked and ready, and when they may be relaxed.

Getting tight for each lift is slightly different. I discuss how to do this in the sections on proper technique for each lift. Here I'll give a brief example from the squat.

When you set up and get the bar properly positioned on your back, you begin by positioning your feet to lift up on the bar. At that point you take a deep breath and tighten your entire body at the same instant. Your calves should be maximally tight, legs, glutes, abs, back, neck, arms, hands, etc. You try to crush the bar with your grip.

When you apply upward force to lift the bar off the squat rack, every muscle in your body flexed. As you step back from the rack, every muscle group is under tension. This allows you to move through space with the weight on your back while under control.

If any muscle group is relaxed, it is like a leak in a hydraulic system. All the force of the weight quickly rushes to the weak spot. If your abs are relaxed, you will collapse forward. If your back is relaxed, you will lose control backward. You get the idea.

Breathing plays a huge role in getting and keeping maximum body tension.

At the most elementary level, every powerlifter knows that before lifting a heavy weight, you inhale and hold your breath. You then hold your breath throughout the lift, or your body relaxes and with reduced body tension, the weight comes crashing down.

Using proper breathing techniques combined with muscle tension can amplify your strength dramatically. You begin by utilizing the lower part of your lungs to create a rock solid mid-section.

When most people take a deep breath, they fill the top part of their lungs and tend to ignore the lower part. You must consciously fill the lower part of your lungs first so that you feel the pressure in your abdomen.

"Belly breathing" is always taught in such diverse sports as the martial arts and distance running. Creating back pressure in your abdomen is the way to absorb a punch, and for distance runners the way to increase oxygen absorption when getting fatigued. In powerlifting, belly breathing allows you to create a rock solid core push that really helps move big iron.

When you get tight, you should think of putting yourself into your most *powerful configuration*. That is, your body is arranged to exert maximum force.

To get into your most powerful configuration, the image you should have in your mind is that you are pulling "into yourself". Fill your lungs with air and hold it. Then pull your shoulders down while flexing your back, pull your quads up, tighten your abs, squeeze your glutes together, and become rigid.

Do NOT suck your stomach in. You should have a flat stomach and a flat back. This posture will allow for generating maximum force.

Your lower lungs should be full of air and creating pressure on your abdominal muscles. This inter abdominal pressure will make your core a totally solid base from which to push.

If you are standing up, this would be how you should feel as you are about to squat.

Each of the powerlifts has specific variations on how you achieve maximum muscle recruitment, proper breathing and body tightness. I'll discuss these in the sections on how to perform each lift.

For now, understand that you need to practice and perfect the principles of recruitment, breathing and tightness on a regular basis.

If you want to excel, you need to *master* these techniques, not merely flip through them occasionally. Practicing them a few times will give you a very modest benefit. Practicing them constantly will give you a huge benefit, and allow you to perform at or near your biological maximum lifts.

Ability to put out 100% effort for one rep

Most people who train with weights have never trained in a way that would allow them to put out 100% of their biological maximum for a single repetition. Conventional fitness training uses higher repetitions and sub-maximal exertion. This is basically endurance type training.

When a lifter does a set of ten repetitions, any one of the reps may only take 60% of his or her maximum effort. Even when people "try their max" in a given lift, they won't have the developed the skill of putting out near 100% of their biological potential.

Learning to put out maximum force for a single repetition means training your central nervous system to send signals to your muscles to contract at the limit of their capability. When done right, it should feel like you are pushing as hard as you possibly can…then adding 10% more. If feels like your body would explode if you relaxed under this level of tension.

While this may sound scary at first, I should remind you that this is one of the skills of strength that is developed by constant and consistent practice. If you work at developing this skill, it will seem automatic and quite "normal".

The issue here is not attitude or the amount of effort expended, it is that training to put out a 100% effort on a single rep is a skill that has to be learned and developed through training.

Be clear about the distinction between training maximum power output and training for endurance. Think of the runners who train for the 100-meter dash and those who train for marathons. Sprinters train for maximum power output and marathon runners train for endurance.

Powerlifters prepare for putting out maximum force for a single rep. Using high rep training will teach your muscles to put out reduced force. A rule for power training is *never do more than 5 reps.* Frequently you will do less than 5 reps. Doing low reps will help train your nervous system to exert a much higher percentage of your maximum capability than high rep sets.

Another thing you should never do is train "to failure". While popular in bodybuilding, this practice will teach your muscles and brain to run a marathon when you are trying to do your best on a 40-yard dash.

How do you develop the skill to put out maximum force for a single rep?

One of the most effective ways to begin training to put out 100% effort is when doing an exercise with a moderate to heavy weight, *move the weight as fast as you can while keeping perfect form.*

When you try to move a heavy lift as fast as you can, the weight may not *actually* move very fast, but it will be moving as fast as you can move it. That is 100% effort.

Mental focus and powerful intention can make a serious difference in how much force you generate every time you lift a weight. When you decide to be powerful, one of the first things you should do is treat every lift as if it were a personal challenge from gravity. Rather than merely "lift" the bar, you are going to "overpower the bar". Instead of simply moving it, you are going to *throw it* (while using perfect technique).

Being mentally aggressive will help you put full force into your lifting instead of merely "doing some reps". Every time you grab a weight, your mind says "I'm going to blast this thing up!!" This is not the stupid screaming and faux intensity you occasionally see from some of the dimmer bulbs in gyms. Rather it is you focusing your full intensity on driving the weight up. You are not just coping with gravity; you are going to kick its ass!

Regular practice of these habits will train you to put out amazing levels of force. Doing the workouts will build your base strength so that you can lift bigger and bigger weights.

There is one advanced training protocol that will help you after you have a solid command of balance, the skill of recruitment and getting tight.

A great *training system* that develops the ability to put out 100% and more is to practice *isometric lifting.* This is a largely forgotten technique that burst on the Olympic Lifting scene around 1960. Although it produced great results, it did not have enough "action" for most Olympic style lifters. I used isometrics back in the early 1960's and have developed a powerlifting program included in this book as Chapter 11.

Regular practice of isometrics can train you to exert maximum force better than anything else I have encountered in 60 years of lifting. I have an array of isometric movements for each of the power lifts that can really help your power output.

Summary

To be able to lift at your maximum capacity you need to develop and perfect several athletic skills unique to powerlifting. First of all, you need to develop good balance and the ability to control heavy weights in space. With a solid base, you need to develop the skills of recruiting every muscle in your body to lift a weight. This involves developing the skills of getting and staying tight and training your central nervous system to put out the maximum power your body is capable of generating.

Perfect form: the key to becoming the strongest you can be

Many lifters are unaware of how vital good technique is to reaching their full potential, so they don't always mine this rich vein. Perfect form is one of those things that may seem relatively less important than some other aspects of training. However, as I'll show you, if you practice perfect form on every rep you do in training, you will have the opportunity to see how good you can become.

The reason it is important to have perfect lifting form is not "style points", but the fact that lifting using perfect form means you get *maximum mechanical advantage*, and *you develop the skill to generate maximum power output doing contest legal lifts.*

Your goal is to be the best lifter you can be, whether you compete or not. Thus, it makes NO sense to do things in your workout that will limit how well you can do on any given day, or place an artificially low ceiling on your ultimate potential.

The technique I see most people using on "gym lifts" really limits how far they can go. Poor technique means people lift far less than they could *on that day,* and prevent them from making any real progress from one month (or year) to the next.

What I'm calling "technique" or "form" are the mechanics of how you perform a lift. There is a huge amount of detail in doing a lift properly. In the chapters on squat, bench press and deadlift I devote 10 to 15 pages detailing how to do a proper lift.

Mastering each of the lifts, and getting close to your full potential requires constant attention to *perfecting your lifting technique.* Mastering proper powerlifting technique is every bit as difficult as mastering the skills for platform diving.

It may *seem* that lifting technique is fairly simple. Remember, the impact of technique is not easily observable because it takes place *inside the body.* In reality, technique has just as much impact on performance as it does in any complex and difficult physical activity.

This idea is very poorly understood. The net effect is that few lifters devote enough attention to *perfecting* their lifting technique. If you want to reach your maximum potential, then consider perfecting your lifting technique as *absolutely critical.*

It may help to think of it this way. For a moment imagine that instead of lifting weights, you were practicing platform diving from the 10-meter board. If you completely ignore working on proper technique, you will never become a very good diver. However, even if you have perfect technique, you will land in the water at the same time you would if you simply fell off the diving platform. If your goal is only to land in the water, any technique is good enough.

Why does perfecting technique work? Because you learn how to use *maximum mechanical advantage when doing a lift.*

What do you do to develop outstanding lifting technique?

The simple answer is: *practice!*

Being an astute reader, you will immediately ask: "practice *what*"?

Obviously, you will practice the athletic skills needed to excel. The big payoff comes when you integrate these skills with perfect lifting technique.

The proper way to do each lift is explained in great detail in the chapters immediately preceding training programs for the squat, bench press and deadlift. Develop excellent lifting technique and you will amaze yourself and others with your performance.

But, developing outstanding technique only happens if you practice (train) a certain way. You can't develop great skill with sloppy practice habits. Thus, here are some little known things about *how* you practice that make a *huge* difference in your eventual accomplishments.

First and foremost, you <u>should *always do every rep of every power lift, regardless of weight, with exactly the same technique.*</u>

You should always strive to do your lightest warm up and your heaviest lift with the same perfect technique. If you do this, whenever you do one of the power lifts, your body will always respond by doing things right. When you set up to do a squat, *your brain has one program set up to do "squat"*. It is the same whether you are doing 135 lbs or 535 lbs.

The great lifters train this way, so it stands to reason that using this approach can have great benefit for anyone who intends to improve their strength.

There are additional reasons why emphasizing perfect technique on every rep is really important. The first is that if you start getting sloppy, you will begin to *practice and perfect your <u>mistakes</u>.*

Many lifters have a consistent flaw in the way they do a lift. When they practice with this flaw in place, they lock in a bad habit. If they are going to correct the flaw, they have to consistently practice with perfect technique. Consistent practice means doing the lift correctly all the time.

Consistently using bad form is one way to insure that progress stops at an artificially low plateau. Having *inconsistent form* is another way to insure that one never gets close to their real potential.

Think about basic skills such as the golf swing or the baseball batting swing. If you have watched lots of amateur players, you will notice that many of them have significant flaws in their swing. However, when they go to "practice" they take a long time doing bad swings while they "warm up". "Getting in the groove" takes a lot of effort, and they readily admit that they do warm ups in a way far different than when they would be swinging "for real".

Among other things, doing a bad swing multiple times means your brain has almost no idea what a good swing is. Since there is no consistency, they are always hunting for the "right feel". By doing bad swing over and over, they "master" doing bad swings.

Using inconsistent technique creates a situation where you never really know whether you are doing a lift properly or not. Each time you do a lift, you have to *think* about doing it correctly. This usually produces inconsistent and baffling results.

If you intend to compete, you must remember that in the stress of a contest situation, your body will automatically do what you have *practiced*. If you have dreadful form during practice, you will revert to dreadful or inconsistent form in a contest.

If you do a lift differently every time, you are always going to feel uncertain about such key things as proper depth in the squat, or proper pausing during the bench press, and many other things that go into executing very complex lifts under maximum load. This is "Death Valley" for competitive lifting.

Some years ago I trained with a group of lifters who generally paid little attention to doing contest legal squats during practice. When we lifted in a contest we were constantly trying to figure out proper squat depth. Our lifting mechanics changed from one attempt to the next. In short, we were at a serious disadvantage before even walking onto the lifting platform for our first attempts. This is an example of a lesson I learned the hard way.

The moral of the story is that if you don't practice perfect technique, when you get to a contest, you will not be able to come close to your full potential because in order to get a lift passed by the referees, you will have to use a much lighter weight than you would if you practiced with perfect form.

Sloppy technique breeds a lot of bad training habits that will undermine any chance a lifter has for long term success. Remember, good technique is designed for maximum mechanical advantage.

Perhaps the most common example of using "poor form" or "bad lifting technique" is the practice of "cheating" when doing a lift. This means that the lifter does one (or more) of the following: does not perform the full range of motion for the lift; alters the mechanics of the lift; or uses extra body movement to complete the lift.

"Cheating" is a common practice in bodybuilding as a way to grind out extra repetitions when the lifter is nearing failure in a given lift. It is a deadly practice if you are trying to build strength because it will subvert building the critical skills of strength discussed earlier. Let me explain.

The practice of not completing the full range of motion for a lift will create systematic weakness in the part of the lift the lifter avoids doing. Usually the part of the lift that is omitted will be the most difficult part. The most common example is not going below parallel in the squat. If a lifter always cheats on squats by "cutting them high", they never train their glutes and hamstrings to contract maximally to bring them "out of the hole" (below parallel).

Altering the mechanics of a lift to get past sticking points is another form of cheating. One of the most common practices is for lifters to raise their butt off the bench to get past the sticking point of the bench press. This distorts the lift in such a way that the lifter systematically weakens their ability to do correct bench presses.

If a lifter does "touch and go" bench presses, they never develop the support muscle strength needed to stabilize the weight on the chest, or the explosive power to drive the weight off the chest after a pause.

Other common examples of distorting the mechanics of a lift are using a double knee bend in a deadlift pull, or resting the bar on the thighs when pulling the deadlift toward lock out.

The third common form of cheating is to introduce extra body movement to move a lift when it gets heavy. Examples of this include bouncing the weight off the chest in the bench press, "touch and go" style bench pressing, "hitching" in the deadlift, bouncing out of the bottom in a squat, or arching the butt off the bench as soon as the bench press bar touches the chest.

The common thing about all of these cheating practices is that they prevent the lifter from staying tight and fully recruiting all their muscles into a lift. The lifter never trains to put out 100% power because they are using the cheat move to substitute for putting full power. In short, cheating will prevent a lifter from *being able to fully develop the critical skills of strength*.

A serious problem with cheating is that in the short run it may give the illusion that the lifter is getting strong. However, progress quickly stalls as cheating will not only retard the development of the key skills noted above, but will cause the lifter to train with weights too close to their existing maximum.

By working too close to their current maximum lift, they prevent the body from adapting slowly to sub-maximal loads, and they *stop making progress.* Over the years I have spent in many different gyms, I am struck by how common it is to see lifters who never improve. They will be lifting exactly the same weight (or slightly less) a year from now, or two years, etc. as they are today.

For lifters who aspire to competing be warned that cheating creates the illusion that the lifter can do contest legal lifts with much heavier weights than they can actually manage when performing in front of judges in a contest. Keep the form strict and regular progress will be the reward.

One final word about "cheating".

Being around lifters who cheat in their training can be disorienting. Sometimes they appear to be lifting more than you. However, you should recognize that these lifters are not competing, and many of their achievements are far less impressive than they appear. They may be "sort of" strong, but their training practices often minimize muscle recruitment, subvert body tightness and never train for maximum power output.

Seeing people use bad form and appearing to lift heavy weights can be a psychological problem, because as a lifter you want to lift as much as you can. However, the false comfort of thinking that you can lift more than you actually can do in a contest is really detrimental to practicing what you need to do in order to improve. Being "real" about the actual lifts that you can handle with perfect form is something you will have to discipline yourself to accept. In the long run, you will benefit greatly by doing this.

The "gym culture" is one that seems to promote exaggeration. Other than filing income taxes, there are few places where so many people take liberties with the facts more consistently than in weightlifting. (I suspect some golfers would argue this point).

You have doubtless met dozens of people who boast about doing really big lifts. These "big lifts" are always done in a gym with only their friends to vouch for them. Usually these grand lifts occurred at some time in the past when the person was "in really good shape".

As you know, a lot of these claims are ridiculous. Often the people who make these claims don't know they are absurd, but often they just want to try to make themselves look good. As a rule of thumb, as a powerlifter, all your personal best lifts should be the ones you have done in a contest. The *real* lifters will respect you for this. You really don't care about the others opinions.

In short, to be the best lifter you can be, treat the following guidance as if it were chiseled in stone:

1. Whenever you do one of the powerlifts, regardless of the weight on the bar, <u>you will always do it in strict accordance with competition rules.</u>
2. Whenever you do one of the powerlifts, regardless of the weight on the bar, <u>you will do it with exactly the same form as nearly perfect as possible.</u>

For example, this means that when you do your bench press warm ups you use the same precise technique (and tightness) as you would if you were doing a competition lift. You will also use perfect technique on every rep of every lift.

Conclusion

Mastering a skill takes a lot of practice. The key thing is to *start practicing and keep practicing*. You will find that your skill builds gradually but consistently.

As you read in the sections that follow, becoming an elite performer in anything never happens overnight. Those who are persistent will always achieve much more than those who quickly tire of trying to improve.

Now let me introduce you to the issues around sport specific conditioning for powerlifting.

Chapter 3

Sport Specific Conditioning: An Overlooked Factor

Conditioning needed by elite performers in different sports is drastically different one from another. Elite distance runners will have a totally different conditioning profile than elite level tennis players, or golfers, or Olympic style weightlifters. It is the same with powerlifting.

Most lifters may be puzzled by the idea that there are sport specific conditioning requirements for powerlifters. However, I believe that this often overlooked factor may have a great deal to do with long term success in the sport, particularly for doing heavy training over extended periods.

Let me begin by re-stating something that is not immediately obvious, but is at the core of why powerlifters need to pay attention to sport specific conditioning:

Lifting heavy weights is a drastically different activity than lifting light weights.

Let me go back to when I first became aware of the need for specialized powerlifting conditioning.

Back in the 1990's my professional life was extremely busy and I was traveling a great deal. By the mid-90's I was flying to Russia and Ukraine on a regular basis, with plenty of long domestic trips thrown in.

I did my best to train regularly, but found that the jumping across a lot of time zones, changing sleep patterns, and irregular eating took a toll. At one point, I had a window of about two months when I would be close to home and could prepare for a contest.

I began my preparations with a plan to do a quick peaking cycle. To my surprise, I found that even though I believed I was in pretty good shape for lifting, my body felt like I was going to break under the work load. I had muscle pains in places I never thought about. My traps and right leg always felt like something was going to rupture.

Weights that I thought I should handle with relative ease seemed to weigh much more. I had trouble going deep in the squat without every alarm bell in my head going off.

Simply being "out of shape"? Yes…but….

It was being out of shape in a very specific way. I could lift *light* weights all day and feel great. It was lifting *heavy training* weights that put me in harm's way.

I struggled through my preparation training and did the meet. My results were pretty modest, but I was always on the brink of pulling a back or leg muscle.

For the next few years I continued to travel a lot, train while on the road, and compete when I could. I noticed that every time I decided to prepare for a contest, it took me at least a month to get "in condition" to do the heavy training for the meet.

Then I saw one of my friends who had been a very prominent lifter try to get back in shape to compete after a long layoff. He worked hard on getting back to heavy lifting for about two months, then suffered a significant leg injury. He had planned a serious come back from being out of the sport for four years, and was stopped cold by a series of minor muscle injuries.

Later, I saw this same thing happen to another lifter friend attempting to come back after a long layoff.

What was the common thread in these cases? Not being "in condition" to do the heavy training associated with powerlifting. We could do light training all day…but the heavy training caused a variety of significant injuries.

This led me to ask what does being "out of shape for heavy lifting *really mean?*"

After considerable reflection and research, I concluded that NOT being in condition to lift heavy weights means: *weakness in the large number of muscles needed to support and stabilize the body wile lifting heavy weights. Many of these muscles are not strong enough to do the work needed. In addition, these muscles are not prepared to work in a coordinated manner while lifting a heavy weight.*

When I had problems, it was always the "small" muscles that were not up to the task. When I saw friends have injuries, it was never the big muscles that were a problem, it was the stabilizers that failed.

Lifting heavy weights requires *full body control.* If the stabilizer muscles are weak or inactive, the lifter does not have the ability to control a big weight. Controlling big weights in space is one of the main things you do in powerlifting.

The stabilizers will not get strong or even be involved while lifting light weights. They are not needed until the weight is formidable. Then, if demands are placed on them, they are not up to the task and likely to fail.

I knew a lifter who had almost limitless potential. However, he never realized a small fraction of his potential because he was *always injured.* He rarely competed, and when he did so, his lifts reflected that he was "just coming back from an injury".

If you are going to realize your full potential, you need to do everything you can to prevent getting injured.   Injuries are not something that just "happen" to you.   Almost all injuries occur because the lifter was not adequately conditioned to do the lift that caused the injury.

Let me do a quick summary of why lifting light weights is so different than lifting heavy weights.

When you lift light weights, most of the muscle activity is *isolation*. You don't need stabilizer muscles for support.

Second, with light weights the tendency is to work *one or two muscle groups at a time*. Because of this, it is very easy to develop muscle imbalances because workouts built on "favorite exercises" don't always involve training opposing muscle groups.

Third, with light weights there is minimal risk to the joints because the level of stress being placed on any given joint is small. There is minimal stress placed on connective tissues with light weights.

Finally, with light weights the issue of controlling the weight in space is negligible. Because the weight is light, keeping balance, stabilizing the weight and moving it in the desired arc does not take a lot of effort. In short, few demands are placed on muscular coordination or athletic movement.

Muscles and connective tissues recover quickly from light workouts.

Heavy weights on the other hand present a totally different challenge. With heavy lifts such as the power lifts, *all the muscles in the body have to be recruited.* Stabilizer muscles are *critical* in generating maximum force needed to move the weight.

With heavy weights, muscle imbalances are a big danger because it takes a balanced muscle structure to lift big iron. Weak muscle groups will tend to become injured.

Weak stabilizer muscles put joints under very high stress when lifting big. Risk to joints becomes extreme because the stresses may be overwhelming.

The stress on connective tissues (tendons and ligaments) can be extreme. Connective tissues adapt to the stresses of heavy lifting more slowly than muscle tissue. Thus, it is possible to injure tendons and ligaments because the muscles capacity for handling big weights grows more rapidly than the connective tissue capacity.

Controlling the weight in space is a significant problem with heavy weights. The need for all muscle groups to work together in a coordinated manner is critical for controlling and moving a big weight.

Recovery from heavy workouts can take much more time than recovery from light workouts. The issue is the extreme intensity of the training as opposed to simply the volume of training.

In a word, muscles must be very <u>resilient</u> to lift heavy weights.

Thus, sport specific conditioning needed for lifting heavy must insure that there are minimal muscle imbalances, build strong stabilizer muscles, and insure that the muscles will work together in a coordinated manner under heavy loads. Furthermore, the muscles and connective tissues must be resilient enough to handle heavy training over weeks and months.

To address this problem, I have identified three types of sport specific conditioning that in my view every lifter should be practicing:

- Core conditioning
- Joint Stability
- Correcting muscle imbalances

Core Conditioning

Two of the three powerlifts are done while standing on your feet. When lifting heavy while standing, a huge burden is placed on the core (abdominals, oblique's, and lower back) for stabilizing and supporting the weight. The core is also intimately involved in generating maximum body power output.

Any lifter who has a lot of body strength has a powerful core.

While the core is critical to optimal athletic performance in *any* sport, the type of core conditioning that golfers will do as opposed to ice skaters as opposed to sprinters is different one from the other.

For powerlifters the type of core conditioning will revolve around supporting huge weights on their shoulders (for the squat), coordinated pulling big weights in the deadlift, and mobilizing all the muscles in the body to push in the bench press.

If some part of the core is weak, squatting with perfect technique becomes nearly impossible. If the lower back is weak, the deadlift is a high risk move. If the core is weak on the bench press, the lifter can't mobilize the strength in the legs, back and abs.

The type of conditioning required is to build the muscular endurance in the core needed to do a lot of heavy training.

Joint Stability

Just about everyone has some part of their anatomy that is more prone to injury issues than another. If you have been training for any period of time, you will no doubt have some recurring issues with a part of your body that gives you problems on a regular basis.

The most common "weak links" are:

- Lower back
- Shoulders
- Knees
- Neck

It is imperative that you take steps to strengthen any "weak link" to reduce the chances of injury that disrupts your training.

Muscle Imbalances

Distortions of the proper alignment of our body come about as a consequence of habitual patterns of over using one set of muscles and under using others. To function properly, bodies must have sets of muscles counter balancing each other. Over developing one set and under using the opposite set lead to structural distortions and thus problems such as bad back, shoulder pain, etc.

These imbalances come about from regularly using or developing muscles unevenly. An example would be a weightlifter who devotes excessive time doing bench presses while paying little attention to developing their back muscles. The muscles on the front become strong and short, while those on the back become long and weak.

Habitual patterns of unbalanced muscle use both causes problems such as back pain, knee pain, etc. and creates the potential for significant injury when weak muscles fail under stress.

To minimize the chance for injury or developing chronic conditions, it is imperative that lifters over age 50 take steps to correct any muscle imbalances they may have developed. While younger lifters will have imbalances, older lifters will usually have accumulated many more years of uneven use. thus, more chance of problems.

In my lifting career, I found that most often weak links occur because some *support muscle* groups were poorly developed, and others over developed. This creates what are known as "muscle imbalances" where one set of muscles creates excessive pull against a much weaker opposing set. The result is often chronic pain, recurring injury or progressive degeneration.

To understand this problem, recognize that for us humans to move, it is necessary to have sets of muscles that pull our bones in one direction or another. There must be one set to move in one direction, and another set to move the other way. For example, the biceps muscle in the arm pulls the arm up and in. The triceps muscle works in the opposite direction, pulling the arm down and back. The two work together.

When muscles develop so that one set is overly strong and the other relatively weak, the skeletal system is pulled out of proper alignment and problems occur. Let me give you a personal example that will show how muscle imbalance can create significant problems for an athlete.

Lower back problems occur with astonishing regularity, particularly for men. Back in the 1980's I was being treated for a chronic low back problem at the University of Washington Hospital. At that time, I was doing competitive running as my primary sport, and did only minimal weight training.

During the rehab portion of the treatment, one of the doctors told me that roughly 80% of men over the age of 40 will have lower back problems. The main cause was that as we age, our abdominal muscles weaken, and our hamstrings get shorter. (This is a chronic problem for runners). Because the abdominals are weak, and the psoas and hamstrings are very powerful, the spine is pulled out of proper alignment, and several nerves can be pinched. The consequence is chronic low back pain.

The most effective treatment for this chronic condition is very straightforward: strengthen the abdominal muscles and stretch the hamstrings. Once I began regular ab work, along with stretching my hamstrings, my back problems disappeared…and have never recurred in the 35 years since my treatment at the UW hospital.

Decades later, it is widely recognized that poor body alignment can cause huge difficulties for any athlete (and regular person). Most physical therapists, sports medicine practitioners and sports trainers recognize the most common (and correctable) source of low back problems.

You don't want to have to go to a therapist for a back problem. Because you are such a wise and clever athlete, you will always be happy to include abdominal work in your workouts. Done on a regular basis, ab work can be your biggest insurance policy against low back problems.

But, you need to expend most of your training time and energy on building strength and power. To do this you can't be doing forty different "rehab-prehab" movements. I have found that there are a few training movements that can work effectively to correct variety of weak links. These can be done at the end of your regular workout with a minimal expenditure of time and energy.

Powerlifting Specific Conditioning Training

Staying injury free when training with heavy weights can be a tall order. However, I have found that there are some training approaches that can address a series of weak links by reducing muscle imbalances, enhancing strength in different ranges of motion, and enhancing overall flexibility.

These training techniques promote whole body conditioning, and if done right will make you highly resistant to muscle tears, failure of support muscles, or weak connective tissues.

The type of whole body conditioning you need as a powerlifter is the sort that doesn't take a lot of time or energy. Let me share a personal anecdote that I think you may find helpful.

In the first fifteen years of my powerlifting career, I occasionally struggled with injuries during training. I thought I had a chronic weakness in my upper trapezius muscle, a problem in my right shoulder, and recurring tendonitis in two different places.

In 2002 I happened to read an article in *Powerlifting USA* about a Russian Special Forces trainer who had come to the US and was introducing (re-introducing) kettlebells to the fitness and weightlifting community. Pavel Tsatsouline (better known simply as "Pavel") was showing how the Russians used a "cannonball with a handle" to forge powerful and resilient bodies.

I remembered kettlebells from my teen age years training with weights. Back in the late 50's weightlifting was not widespread, and gyms were few and far between. The gyms that were around always seemed to have some training tools that dated back to the old time strong men. Kettlebells were among the tools that the old timers used regularly. This was long before the first "machine" made an appearance in a gym.

I have long believed that a lot of the best and most effective training devices were "old school". So, when kettlebells suddenly appeared again, I instantly bought a set of three from the new Russian capitalist. The weights were 16, 24 and 32 kilos (35, 53 and 70 pounds).

I began training with these delightfully sinister looking devices immediately. Because I was already a competitive powerlifter, I progressed quickly. Because no one told me otherwise, I trained myself to do the one hand kettlebell snatch using Pavel's written instructions. These days you can usually find a qualified kettlebell instructor who can teach you how to do this deceptively difficult move. However, if you are determined, you can learn it on your own.

The bottom line for me was that in I developed a nearly bulletproof core, eliminated any joint pain, my trap problem vanished, and my shoulder problem went away. Furthermore, I developed overall resilience that kept me injury free in another decade of heavy training and competitive powerlifting.

All this happened to me when I was in my 60's. That is the age when a person is supposed to be getting more vulnerable rather than bulletproof.

During the same time period, several of the lifters with whom I had regular contact suffered significant injuries that kept them from training for extended periods. Two suffered career ending injuries. While I can't be certain, my long experience in training tells me that the lifters who sustained injuries had good strength, but also had muscle imbalances, limited flexibility, and lacked the resilience needed for extended hard training.

In short, I believe *selective* training with kettlebells are the best overall way to build and keep a powerful resilient body.

What do I mean by *selective*?

My approach is to pick a few kettlebell exercises that give you the most "bang for the buck". You are not trying to compete in the Cross-Fit Games, your goal is to condition the vulnerable links in your power chain.

To that end, I recommend that you *master* a few key movements that IMHO will do great things for you.

If you don't have access to kettlebells, these movements can all be done with dumbbells. Depending on the type of dumbbells you have, the grip may require some ingenuity.

Powerlifting Specific Conditioning Training Routine

The five exercises described below should be done at the end of your regular workouts. Use weights that are relatively easy for you to do. The most important impact of this program is the *cumulative training effect* of doing this training over a long period of time. You are not aiming for a "PR" in each lift, but rather you want the *resilience* that comes from consistent practice over weeks, months and years.

I have listed some kettlebell exercises as assistance work in the sections on each lift. Occasionally, the lifts included in the assistance work will be the same as in the conditioning drills. If you do the lift once in a training session that will be sufficient.

Perform the conditioning routine after each "heavy day" training session. Do **two sets** of each exercise. The number of reps will vary with each of the exercises.

Movement #1 – Kettlebell Swing – (Russian Style)

The kettlebell swing is the basis for building strength and resilience in the glutes, hamstrings, lower back, shoulders, hips and (*very important*) the abdominal muscles. It is also the basis for all the more advanced kettlebell movements.

There are two versions of the swing. One is the Russian style where the weight is brought up until your arms are *parallel* to the floor. The other is the Cross-Fit style swing. In this version, you raise the kettlebell until your arms are just short of being directly overhead. These are basically two different exercises, but they are both called the swing. This causes considerable confusion.

I suggest you use the Russian style swing where your arms only go to parallel with the floor.

The movement begins by swinging the bell back between your legs as if you were hiking a football. If you never hiked a football, just swing the kettlebell back between your legs and bend your knees so that your arms extend behind you as shown.

Your weight should be on your heels as you swing the weight back. Your head should be up and your eyes looking straight ahead. Your arms should only be used to hang on to the weight.

When the kettlebell is as far behind you as it is going to go, drive your hips forward explosively and straighten your legs. This force should propel the kettlebell upward to a position where your arms are parallel to the floor. Don't apply any force with your arms. All the power comes from your glutes, hamstrings and abs.

You know you are doing this movement correctly when you feel the force in your abs.

When the kettlebell becomes "weightless" with your arms parallel to the floor, allow it to swing back to the position where it is between your legs, and do another rep.

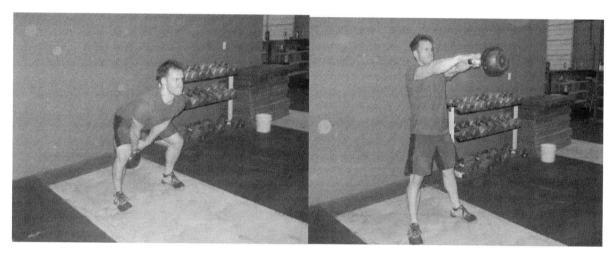

Swing position back between legs   Swing position with arms parallel to floor

Movement #2 – One hand snatch

This is one of the greatest single exercises ever invented. Pavel called this "The Tsar of all Exercises". The one hand snatch is technically very difficult to master, but you should dedicate yourself to learning how to do this movement correctly. It will pay you huge dividends.

Doing a few sets of one hand snatches at the end of your workout will pay huge dividends in terms of strengthening your abdominal core, as well as your hips, back and legs. Your arms, upper back and shoulders will also benefit tremendously. The snatch is an athletically demanding movement that will enhance your balance, explosive power and endurance.

Why if it is such a great exercise do so few people do it? Very simple....it is *hard!* This is *not* one of those "Ken and Barbie" movements.

The kettlebell snatch is one of the great movements in strength and power. It is part of what I call "the great tradition" of strong men and women. Every time you grasp a kettlebell to do a snatch, feel the power of the thousands of strong athletes who have done this almost mystical movement. When you do the snatch regularly, you join this tradition.

The kettlebell snatch is one of the greatest single exercises ever invented. Pavel called this "The Tsar of all Exercises". Be advised that the one hand kettlebell snatch is technically very difficult to master. For this reason, I suggest that you may want to begin doing one handed snatches with a dumbbell.

The biggest difference between the dumbbell and kettlebell versions of the one hand snatch is that the weight of the dumbbell is always in the center of your hand. Because the bulk of the kettlebell is outside your hand, you have to move your hand around the flying weight or it will flip over and blast you on your forearm. This can be very painful, and can be dangerous.

The main difficulty of trying to learn the movement from a book is getting the subtle hand move down where at the top of the lift you slip your hand behind the kettlebell rather than have it flip over and hit your forearm.

Pay particular attention to the hand positioning and practice with a light weight to get the technique correct.

The one hand kettlebell snatch begins by swinging the weight back between your legs, and propelling it up by quickly driving your hips forward and explosively straightening your legs. The drive from your hips and legs should propel the weight upward.

All the force that drives the weight overhead will come from your hips, abs and legs. You begin accelerating the weight forward when your arm has reached the full backswing position. You should have generated all the force needed to get the weight overhead when your arm is at about a 30-degree angle in front of you.

Other than pulling the weight toward you on the way up, your arms should not be anything other than "ropes" that connect the weight to your body. All of the force that drives the weight overhead should come from snapping your hips forward and straightening your legs quickly.

You should feel the pull in your abs if your trunk is positioned correctly. If you feel it in your lower back, you are

The picture below shows how you should pull the weight toward you as you drive the weight upward. Your arm should not be fully extended, but rather pulling the weight back toward you. The idea is to minimize the arc that the weight travels when you pull it upward. Limiting the arc on the upward pull gives you the most efficient use of power when lifting the weight.

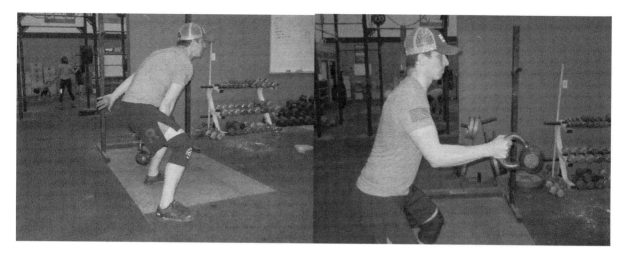

Swing back between legs

Pull the weight toward you on the way up

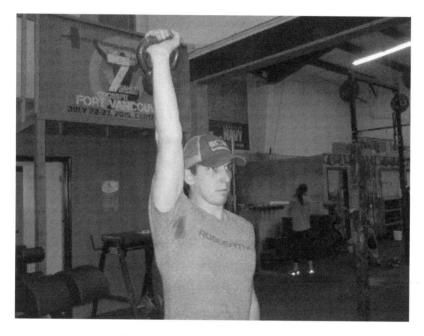

Finish positon at full lock out

It is important that you have the palm of your hand turned toward outward as you begin the upward swing. That is if you are holding the weight with your right hand, your palm should be facing your right leg as you begin the upward acceleration.

By keeping your palm facing outward at the bottom of the snatch, your hand will naturally rotate to a palm forward position as the weight travels overhead. This keeps the kettlebell from flipping over your hand and smashing your forearm.

You are going to try and make the weight travel straight upward in front of you, as that is the most efficient path. To do this keep your weight back on your heels and pull back as the weight accelerates upward. As I said, you want to minimize the arc.

This part of the snatch movement is sometimes described as "pull" that is immediately followed by "punch" as the weight is locked out overhead. When the weight is locked out at arm's length, your palm should be facing forward.

At this point, drop the weight straight down and swing it back between your legs for another rep.

To get the technique down it is advisable that you begin with a weight you can handle easily for ten reps. Over time you will increase the weight. Eventually, you should learn how to do this movement with a kettlebell as it is one of those truly great exercise movements that have huge benefit for your whole body.

If the snatch is such a great exercise, why do so few people do it? Very simple....it is *hard!* This is *not* one of those "Ken and Barbie" movements.

The kettlebell snatch is one of the great movements in strength and power. It is part of "the great tradition" of strong men and women. Every time you grasp a kettlebell to do a snatch, feel the power of the thousands of strong athletes who have done this almost mystical movement. *You* are now joining this tradition.

Movement #3- Two hand kettlebell clean and press

Standing dumbbell or kettlebell presses are another body power builder that has few rivals. This will work all your upper body, as well as your abs, hips, and legs. It is an athletically demanding lift that can help teach you to mobilize your body force to drive the weight overhead.

Standing presses are a "whole body" lift. You can use them to learn how to tighten your entire body, and then drive the weight upward.

In both the dumbbell press and the kettlebell press, you will begin by bringing the weights to your shoulders (the "clean"). At that point your entire body should be completely rigid. Squeeze the handles as hard as you can, and with your legs, abs, glutes and back completely locked down tight, drive the weights overhead.

You should concentrate on recruiting as many muscles as you can to grind the weight up to arm's length. To be useful to you, these presses must be a *whole body lift.*

Anyone can do presses with little weights that don't require you to mobilize the whole body into the lift. In your press training, over time you will learn how to focus all your body force into the palm of your hand. This is great training for any pressing movement.

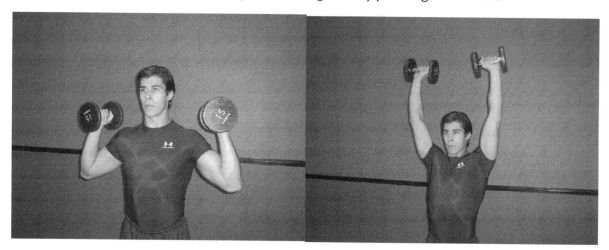

Dumbbell Press – Start **Dumbbell Press - Lockout**

Bring the kettlebells to your shoulders in the position as shown. Your palms will face each other when holding the weights at the shoulders. This is called the "rack" position. As you drive the weight overhead your palms will rotate until they are facing forward when you complete the lift at full lockout.

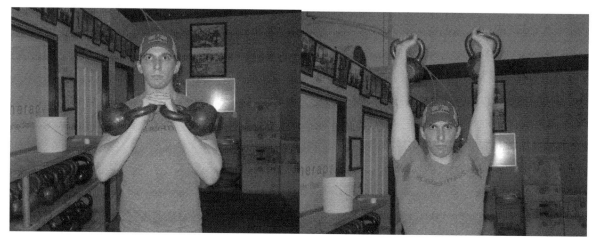

Kettlebell Press – Start **Kettlebell Press - Lockout**

The point of doing overhead presses is to develop the ability to mobilize your body's pressing power, and to develop all the support muscles needed to press effectively.

You should *never* cheat or use poor technique in this lift. You are using this lift to train your central nervous system to get all your muscles involved in the act of pressing.

You will practice pressing by doing two sets of *five reps* in each conditioning training session.

Movement #4 – Overhead Walk

Protecting your shoulders is something you will need to do your entire lifting career. The overhead kettlebell (or dumbbell) walk is a lift devised to strengthen all the support muscles in the shoulder. This helps prevent injury, and strengthens the entire shoulder support system.

This exercise was developed by trainers for teams in the National Football League to help prevent (and also rehabilitate) shoulder injuries. Since first appearing in 2008, this movement has spread to other sports where athletes put a lot of strain on their shoulders. Tennis players, swimmers, baseball players and other athletes are using this very simple movement to help build resilient and healthy shoulders.

The cool thing about this movement is that it is very simple to perform, and it can benefit anyone who wants to protect their shoulders for any type of lifting. The movement is simply while standing, take a dumbbell in one hand, press it to arm's length overhead, and keeping it overhead walk forward between 50 to 100 feet. At that point, switch hands and put the dumbbell overhead with the other hand and walk back the same distance.

Benefits from this movement are that all the muscles that stabilize the shoulder are activated when you walk with the weight overhead. Literally every muscle from the tip of the fingers to the tip of the toes is activated in some degree.

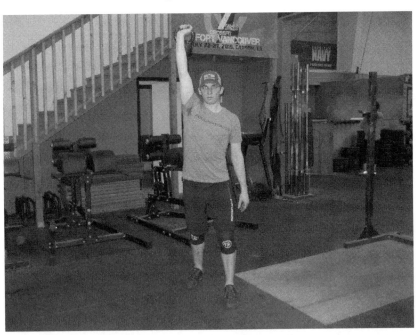

Kettlebell Walk – Hold the weight overhead and walk

It is prudent to begin with a weight that you can handle easily for walks of 70-100 feet. You should begin by doing two circuits with a light dumbbell. You can add one walking circuit each time until you are doing five circuits. At that point you can increase the weight, and drop back to doing two to four circuits. As you get stronger, it will be easier to walk with more weight.

You can vary the intensity of the training by adding more distance to the walk, or using a heavier weight.

This movement can also be used to help rehabilitate shoulders that have been injured. It is advised that if you have a shoulder injury, you be cautious about the amount of weight you use. If your injury is severe, I strongly recommend that you get help from a fully qualified physical therapist.

In your conditioning training you will do one or two circuits each training session.

Movement #5 – Goblet Squat

The goblet squat will work all the support muscles in your body in a coordinated manner. This movement has super conditioning benefits when practiced over extended periods of time. Doing goblet squats will keep your abs well trained for squatting and keep your full range of motion for going low in the barbell squat.

Begin by grasping a kettlebell with both hands by the outside part of the handle. Bring the weight up to your chin area and hold it in place with both hands. The weight will be supported by your arms even though it may touch your chest. Your arms should not touch your knees, nor should you rest the kettlebell on your chest.

Set your feet at the same position you normally plan to use for your competition squat. If you want, you can vary the foot spacing to get slightly different muscle activation patterns.

Keep your head erect, and go down into a deep squat position. Go as deep as you can go while keeping your back flat. Keep your shins vertical during the squat. When you are at the bottom, return to a standing positon. Your arms will support the weight throughout the movement.

Begin using a relatively light weight as the purpose of this drill is to condition support muscles and give you an optimal stretch. As this will be the last exercise you do in your workout, your goal should be to do two good sets, and not worry too much about how much weight you use.

Begin with a modest weight and over a long period of time gradually work up to doing your sets with a 24K to 32K kettlebell depending on your size.

Remember this is a conditioning exercise, not an all-out squat effort.

This exercise is great for building powerful stabilizer muscles, a strong core and great balance. In short, this movement gives a lot of payback for the effort. You also get a great stretch in the hips, glutes and lower back.

You should do **2 sets of 8-10 repetitions** with the goblet squat. As the weight feels lighter, you can add reps up to a maximum of 15.

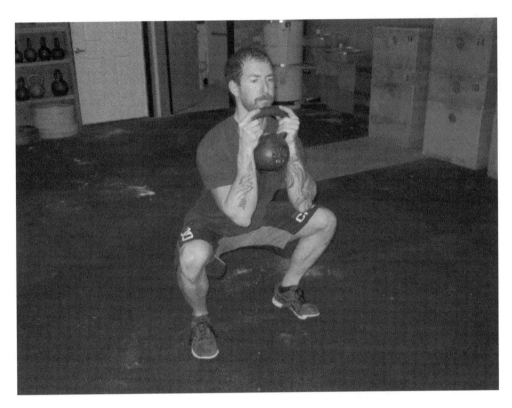

Kettlebell Goblet Squat – Bottom position

Develop the habit of doing conditioning drills every workout, and you will enjoy a much more injury free career.

Chapter 4

Training for Power: Building Training Plans

"If you have no plan, your plan is to fail…."

-Andrew "Bull" Stewart – 11-time world powerlifting champion and *Sports Illustrated* magazine "Athlete of the 20th Century" in Powerlifting

That short quote sums up the importance of training plans. If you have no training plan, you will never come close to achieving your full potential.

In this chapter, I'll show you how to build your own training plan. The format will be designed for a 50-year-old powerlifter, with lots of work, but clearly defined times for recovery.

There are four training days each week. Three of the days will be focused on each power lift: the squat, bench press and deadlift. One of the training days will be "light" and designed to enhance recovery, conditioning, and athletic skill.

All workouts will be done on a 4 to 8-week training cycle. There is a separate cycle for each of the power lifts. Each cycle has a prescribed series of exercises that are to be done with weights you calculate as a percentage of your 1 rep maximum lift.

At the end of the cycle, you will change to a different training cycle. Changing routines is essential in order to continue making progress.

You will select training cycles based on a plan for when you will be competing, or attempting a personal best in a lift. The idea is that all of your training is organized around times when you want to be primed to do your best lifting.

Let me take you through the process of going from a yearly training plan to what do you do *this week*.

Yearly Training Calendar

Powerlifting training will be significantly different for most people than "fitness training" in one major way. <u>The workouts you do will be defined by the dates during the year that you intend to compete.</u>

Training plans are devised to prepare the lifter for competitions that occur during the year. Experienced lifters who compete at a high level will usually compete in *two to four* lifting meets a year. *The entire training schedule is organized around being ready to do their best in those events.*

Some of you may think that competing only two to four times a year does not sound like much. Trust me, doing four powerlifting competitions with the necessary training will be all you can handle.

I can say this from the perspective of having been a competitive runner for 22 years. In some seasons, I would race every two weeks, occasionally more often. The distances I ran were between 10K and 10 miles with an occasional half marathon included. When I say "competitive", I mean that I normally finished in the top 10% of the runners in my age group, occasionally in the top 1%.

Recovery time for a major running competition is measured in days or weeks. In powerlifting, it is measured in weeks and months. The difference is that running is endurance work, and powerlifting is maximum muscle stress. Different stuff….

For the person who does not intend to compete in powerlifting, but wants to do powerlifting training for their own health and fitness, they can select dates during the coming year when they will attempt personal records (PR's). These PR attempt dates can then be used to organize the yearly training calendar.

The cool thing about having a yearly training calendar is that it helps you focus on continuing improvement. The calendar helps define on where you want to be in three months, six months a year, etc.

Here is an example of a yearly training calendar based on the lifter competing in June and December.

> June 1-30 – Conditioning and lifting technique training
> July 1- August 30 – Basic power building cycle
> Sept 1 – Sept 30 – Explosive movements, bands, heavy assistance work
> Oct 1- November 30 – 8 week peaking cycle for Dec 1 competition
> Dec 1 – **Competition**
> Dec 2-31 – Muscle endurance training
> Jan 1- Feb 28 – Enhanced power training
> March 1- 31 Speed training – functional isometrics
> April 1 – 30 –Heavy power rack training
> May 1- 31 – 4 week peaking cycle for June 1 competition
> June 1 – **Competition**

When you make your yearly calendar, begin with the dates you intend to compete and then fill in the cycles you intend to use by working backward to the present.

The four to eight weeks immediately preceding the competition should be a *peaking cycle* for each lift.

Preceding the peaking cycle should be a cycle designed to build speed or explosiveness. The period prior to the peaking cycle must be used to push your strength in very different ways than you use when simply training on full power lifts. That is why I have included partial lifts, explosive strength, isometrics and a range of other challenges that can build your power.

You should select as many cycles as you need to fill your calendar back to the present time.

Some lifters will ask why it is necessary to change the training program every month or two. The physiological reason is called the *principle of adaptation.* In short, it means that your body adapts to the demands of a particular workout in a short period of time. At that point, further adaptation stops.

When adaptation stops, you have to come up with a new challenge, or you stay at the same level or decline slightly.

If you could just keep adapting indefinitely, all you would have to do is lift relatively heavy each time and eventually you would be lifting tons of weight. Your body does not work that way.

Some of you may have heard the story of the ancient Greek strongman Milo. He began lifting a young calf daily, and the theory was that he could keep lifting the animal as it grew and he would eventually be able to lift a giant animal. No way! The calf grows faster than your body can accommodate, and the body quits accommodating new loads pretty rapidly.

For that reason, we change what we do in training every 4 to 8 weeks and allow the body to accommodate to something new.

Different training cycles are designed to stimulate strength development by using different types of exercises, different stresses, speeds, weighs and different combinations of sets and reps.

It is important to understand that you will be selecting specific training cycles for each power lift (squat, bench press and deadlift

When you make a yearlong plan, it is your best estimate at what will work for the coming twelve months. You may need to revise the calendar based on the results of a contest. No problem. But, make your revision based on a systematic appraisal of what you need to do to improve, not on a whim.

While it is true no training program works for very long, it is also true that most programs need to be done to completion to get the desired results.

One thing you should *never do* is change workouts in the middle of a cycle. Once you start a cycle, finish it. If you don't finish the cycle, you throw away any gains you may have made.

Like the examples in the list on how to guarantee failure, one of the habits of lifters who never make progress is they abandon their systematic training plans just because they read an article on some web site or read an article at random that promised miracle gains. These lifters are like hummingbirds going from flower to flower…. never staying with one thing very long, doing a lot of training, but never getting anywhere.

Cycles

If you keep doing the same workout all the time, you will quickly hit a plateau and never improve your strength. The idea behind cycles is to give your body new training challenge on a regular basis so that you can continue to build your strength.

Getting stronger involves training where you begin using weights that are lighter than your maximum and over a period of a few weeks work up to using heavier weights. A cycle is a plan for a series of workouts to be done over a few weeks where you will increase the weight you lift by in a series of planned increases.

In the sections on each lift, I provide five different training cycles each of which gives you a significantly different training challenge than the one preceding it. Doing different things in different combinations is one of the main ways that you improve your strength and skill as a powerlifter.

Cycles are four to eight week groups of exercises. In this book, you will find five training cycles for each of the powerlifts (squat, bench press and deadlift).

Most of the cycle programs included here can be used in any order, just so that you don't repeat one you just finished. The only exception is what is called a "peaking cycle" that is used in the 4-8-week period immediately before a contest or maximum lift attempt.

Your yearly calendar is made up of the cycles you plan to use in the coming 12 months. The next six months should be pretty much cast in stone. The longer term plans can be more flexible.

How do you decide which cycle to use?

If you are just beginning a six-month preparation for a maximum lift, OR you are just starting out in powerlifting, I would recommend that you do your first cycle using the 5 sets – 5 reps format for the primary power lift. You will do this along with the recommended assistance exercises.

The next cycle you select should be significantly different than the one you just completed. If you have been doing 5 x 5, then using the 7 sets of 2 reps would be in order.

In the workout plans for each lift, you will find a variety of cycles. After you develop experience with them, you will be able to devise your own. The key to progress will be to regularly change up what you do.

An example of how to use the calendar to make a training plan

Let's take a hypothetical lifter named James, who will be using the training cycles in this book. Let's say it is now the last week of November, and James wants to enter a contest next June. He wants to get all of his lifts up by that time. The contest is six months from December 1.

To organize his six-month training plan, James would select training cycles for each lift, squat, bench press and deadlift. Let's say he begins with scheduling deadlift training.

His starting point is to go to the date of the contest, let's say June 1, and work backwards to the present date. He starts building his six-month plan by scheduling a peaking cycle in the eight weeks immediately before the contest. That takes all of April and May.

Next he assesses where he is now, and what workouts would have the most potential to help him. He selects the foundation program which emphasizes doing 5 sets of 5 reps of the deadlift along with assistance work. So he plans to do a 5 x 5 cycle for the deadlift beginning on December 1, and continuing for eight weeks.

That would leave the time between the start of the peaking cycle on April 1 and the end of the 5 x 5 cycle on January 31. In other words, February and March.

James decides to include two four week cycles in that period. The first a power rack training cycle and the second a cycle emphasizing use of elastic bands.

At this point, James has planned what training cycles he will use to train for the deadlift for the six months leading up to the contest.

He will then do this same process for the squat and bench press. At the conclusion of that planning, James has laid out all the training he will do for the next six months.

His next task is to plan his weekly training schedule.

His starting point is to decide which lifts to do on which days. Because the squat and deadlift take the most energy and require the most recovery time, he schedules them on Monday and Thursday of each week. He needs at least one full day of recovery before deadlifting, so he schedules his bench press training on Tuesday with Wednesday being a day with no training.

He also wants to have one day to do light training to help with his recovery. He selects Friday for that, with both Saturday and Sunday having no training scheduled at all.

His planned weekly schedule looks like this:

- Monday – **Heavy squat** workout + squat assistance work + conditioning work
- Tuesday – **Heavy bench press** workout + bench press assistance + conditioning
- Wednesday – Rest and recover
- Thursday – **Heavy deadlift** workout + deadlift assistance work + conditioning
- Friday – Light work on all 3 lifts + conditioning
- Saturday – Rest
- Sunday – Rest

Let's assume that James now has a plan for how he will do his training for the June 1 lifting meet. His next task is to fill in *what he will do in each workout.*

That task is straightforward since he has already selected which cycles he will be using. Let's use the 5 x 5 deadlift cycle to show what he will do.

Since every lift he is supposed to do is based on a percentage of his 1 rep maximum lift, he begins by preparing a table showing the actual weights that represent each percentage. His 1 rep maximum won't change during the eight-week cycle, so he only has to make these calculations once.

Determining Your One Rep Maximum Lift

Whenever you select a cycle program, you need to do some numerical calculations, since the squats, bench presses and deadlifts you do will be based on a percentage of your 1 rep maximum lift.

Your one rep maximum lift (1RM) in each of the powerlifts is the basis for developing your personalized training program. If you are an experienced powerlifter, you will know what your 1 rep max is. If this is new to you, here is how you determine this important number.

The most obvious way of defining your 1RM is the most weight you are able to lift <u>with perfect technique</u> for a single rep. I emphasize doing the lift with perfect technique, because counting a lift done with less than contest legal form will not do you any good.

Having been in gyms for over a half century, I can assure you that about 99% of the squats you see in the typical gym and over 99% of the bench presses you see are *not* contest legal. Don't look around and take the haphazard standards of performance to be the technique you need to master.

For example, I have met many gym lifters who claimed to have done a huge bench press who were absolutely crushed with modest weights when they had to pause the bar on the chest. Likewise, I have heard some claims of massive squats that proved to be complete fantasy when the lifter had to go below parallel. I'll save the story of the hapless dork who told me he could deadlift 900 pounds for later.

Unless you already train with competing powerlifters who know what a contest legal lift looks like, you will need to really pay attention to the sections of this book on proper technique for each lift. You must insure that you have an accurate fix on what you can *actually* do for a 1RM.

Starting with a "real" 1RM number will be a great help in the long run. You may begin at a far lower number than you expected...but use it as your *real* starting point and you will be rewarded with consistent progress. If you start with an unrealistically high number, and your progress will stall out quickly and you will be stuck at that level indefinitely.

I don't recommend trying to extrapolate your 1RM from anything other than your best at 2 or 3 reps. If you use any higher number of reps as a basis for extrapolation, the number you get will be way too high.

Once you have established your 1RM, and have a date in the future when you will be doing a contest or attempting a personal best, you are ready to set up your training cycles and make your training plans.

For purposes of this example, let's say that James has best lifts of 400 pounds in the squat, 300 in the bench press and 450 in the deadlift. The following table would show all the relevant weights for each lift as a percentage of his 1 rep maximum.

	Squat	Bench Press	Deadlift
Current 1 RM	400 lbs.	300 lbs	450 lbs
5%	20	15	22.5
50%	200	150	225
60%	240	180	270
70%	280	210	315
80%	320	240	360
90%	360	270	405
100%	400	300	450
105%	420	315	472.5
110%	440	330	495

You will notice that one of the calculations is "5%". Being an astute man, James knows that to estimate a weight that is "65%" of max or some other percentage ending in 5, all he has to do is add the 5% weight to the 60% weight to establish what he will lift.

His next task is to develop a plan for the *actual weights he will use in training for the entire cycle.* This is simpler than it may sound at first, since after making the initial calculation of 1 rep max, all that is required in the example programs below is to add 5 pounds to the squat and bench press each week.

Shown below are two sample eight week plans based on James' current 1 rep max.

Squat: 8-week cycle of 5 x 5   Current 1 rep max = 400 lbs.

	Week 1	Week 2	Week 3	Week 4
Set 1:	5 @ 50% - 200	205	210	215
Set 2:	5 @ 70%- 280	285	290	295
Set 3:	5 @ 80% - 320	325	330	335
Set 4:	5 @ 70% - 280	285	290	295
Set 5:	5 @ 60% - 240	245	250	255

	Week 5	Week 6	Week 7	Week 8
Set 1:	220	225	230	235
Set 2:	300	305	310	315
Set 3:	340	345	350	355
Set 4:	300	305	310	315
Set 5:	260	265	270	275

Assistance work:
    Kettlebell swing: 2 sets 10-15 reps
    Back hyperextension: 2 sets 10 reps
    Hanging leg raise: 2 sets 10-20 reps

Conditioning work:
    Kettlebell swing: (skip – done in assistance work)
    Kettlebell snatch: 2 sets 5 reps
    Dumbbell/Kettlebell clean and press: 2 sets of 5 reps
    Overhead walk: 2 circuits
    Goblet squat: 2 sets 8-10 reps

Bench Press: 8-week cycle of 5 x 2   Current 1 rep max = 300 lbs

	Week 1	Week 2	Week 3	Week 4
Set 1:	2 @ 65% = 195	200	205	210
Set 2:	2 @ 75% = 225	230	235	240
Set 3:	2 @ 85%= 255	260	265	270
Set 4:	2 @ 75%= 225	230	235	240
Set 5:	2 @ 65%= 195	200	205	210

	Week 5	Week 6	Week 7	Week 8
Set 1:	215	220	225	230
Set 2:	245	250	255	260
Set 3:	275	280	285	290
Set 4:	245	250	255	260
Set 5:	215	220	225	230

Assistance work:
- Power cage lock outs
- Incline dumbbell press
- Close grip bench press
- Upright rowing

Conditioning work:
- Kettlebell swing: (skip – done in assistance work)
- Kettlebell snatch: 2 sets 5 reps
- Dumbbell/Kettlebell clean and press: 2 sets of 5 reps
- Overhead walk: 2 circuits
- Goblet squat: 2 sets 8-10 reps

You will notice that the vast majority of the time, the power lifts are done well below 1 rep max. This is because if someone lifts at or near their limit all the time, they never improve. They tend to exhaust themselves almost every training session, and never fully recover.

Think about improving your strength as if you were climbing stairs. At the lowest steps, you have a base level of strength where say you can grind out 5 reps of a lift with 100 pounds. As you climb the stairs, your base strength improves and you find it easy to do 8 reps with the weight that used to be a challenge for 5 reps. Over time your base increases and you find that the old challenge is now easy.

You move up the stairs by working below your maximum. Keep increasing the sub-maximal base strength and your peak strength also keeps increasing.

All of us have been in gyms where you see lifters grinding out reps near their max every training session. What is interesting is that if you come back a year (or two years) later, these lifters are still struggling with the same weights. If someone lifts too close to their maximum all the time, they will stay on a plateau and never improve!

The key to improving is building up your base load of strength, and then gradually improving that base over time. When you go for a peak performance, you start from a higher base, so your peak lift is higher.

Improving your base strength means that weights that were "really heavy" for you in an earlier period are now light. What took a major effort to grind out 4-5 reps is now easily done for 8-10 reps. There is a new upper limit on what you can lift.

What do I do THIS week?

When you have selected a specific program for your training cycle, the first week of the cycle, you will calculate the weights you use based on a percentage of your 1 rep max. For example, if you are doing the 5x5 squat program, the first week you will be doing each of the five sets with the poundage you calculated when you started the cycle.

In the example above, the first set of squats is 50% of James's 1 rep max of 400 pounds which would be 200 pounds. The second set is 60% which is 240 pounds and so forth.

The program calls for a 5-pound increase on each set every week. So, every week, James will increase each of the weights he does by 5 pounds. So the second week his opening set will be at 205 pounds, next set 245, and so forth.

Thus, what James (or you) will do on each of the powerlifts in each workout of the cycle is determined by the calculations done at the start of the cycle.

Then include the assistance exercises that are part of each cycle.

As you can see, there is a *lot* of information to track. This is why I emphasize over and over that keeping written records is *critical*. There is way too much detail to remember. Staying on a plan, and knowing where you at any given time requires accurate records.

It is absolutely imperative that you have written records of all your workouts. You should write them down as you do the training. A simple notebook is sufficient for you to record every set, rep and weight of each exercise you do on each day. You can also use one of the many new software apps that are available. Basically, whatever works best for you.

Why is this so important?

The main reasons are:

- Since you have a <u>written plan,</u> you need to know if you are doing what is in the plan
- If you are having problems, where are they?
- At the end of each training cycle, you need to see what worked for you and what didn't

Never believe that you can rely on your memory. It will *always* be inaccurate. There is way too much detail to remember accurately. In any given week you will do between 80 and 120 individual sets of different exercises most with different weights. In an eight-week training cycle you will do well over 1000 different sets. Think you can (or should) remember each of them?

One of the habits of unsuccessful lifters is that they never keep systematic records. One of the habits of very successful lifters is that they keep good records of their training.

Written records of your training allow you to do an "after action" review of how your training cycle went. What worked and what did not? Did you do too many of one thing, and not enough of another? Do you have a recurring problem in one part of a lift?

"Light" Training Day

If you lift heavy every workout, you will quickly hit a plateau and never progress. If you are going to get stronger, it is imperative that you use your training schedule to facilitate your recovery from heavy lifting.

Having pumped heavy iron for two and a half decades, I'm a big fan of using a training format where you do intense training on each of the three lifts once a week, and a fourth workout where you work on consolidating your gains and general conditioning. The fourth workout where you do a "light" workout helps your muscles to rebuild, and helps train your brain to use perfect form and put out max power.

Remember, bodies over age 50 are capable of some mind blowing feats of strength, but to accomplish this, it is critical not to over train. I keep harping on the need for solid recovery because it is so widely ignored.

It has always amazed me that so many people are ignorant of this fact. Over my half century plus of training in gyms, I have seen thousands of people who insist on training at their limits every workout. They never improve from one year to the next, and eventually begin to regress.

Remember, recovery and consolidation are the way to get strong. Constantly pushing your limits is the way to get tired….and little else.

On light training day, do each of the powerlifts for two sets of five with light weights. I like to say this lifting reminds your body of "all the fun you have doing powerlifting". The key is doing light weights at a relatively high speed. This keeps the central nervous system ready to go hard on the heavy training days, but doesn't over work the muscles so that you won't have recovered by the time the heavy training days come around again.

Next, do a sports specific conditioning routine with dumbbells and kettlebells.

At the conclusion of the session, you should be nice and sweaty, but feel that you could do more. If you conclude the week feeling exhausted, you are going to hit a plateau or get weaker in short order.

1. **Bench Press**

Begin your training session with one warm up set and two training sets of the bench press, both for five repetitions. My rationale for putting the bench press first is that your body may be stiff following heavy deadlift training day, and the bench press eases you into the workout.

> Set 1: Warm up 1 set 5 reps
>
> Set 2: Training set – 5 reps at 50% of 1 rep max
>
> Set 3: Training set – 5 reps at 60% of 1 rep max

Always use perfect technique. Pause the first three reps on the chest, and drive the bar up to lock out quickly. Touch and go for the last two reps.

You should finish this feeling refreshed rather than worked.

2. **Deadlift**

The deadlift comes next on light day. You may be stiff from your previous heavy deadlift day, so this session is aimed at getting you lose and moving the bar quickly.

> Set 1: Warm up – 5 reps
>
> Set 2: Training set – 5 reps at 40% of 1 rep max
>
> Set 3: Training set – 5 reps at 50% of 1 rep max

Concentrate of perfect technique. Focus on recruiting every muscle in the body for the pull. Just because the weight is light, you should not lapse into the bad habit of using only a few muscles to pull.

3. **Squat**

Now that you have done the first two powerlifts, you should be warmed up enough to do light squats with ease.

> Set 1: Wall squats (to insure perfect form) – 5 reps to full depth
>
> Set 2: Training set – 5 reps to maximum depth with 30% of 1 rep max
>
> Set 3: Training set – 5 reps to maximum depth with 40% of 1 rep max

As always, use perfect technique and concentrate on recruiting all the muscles in your body to move the squat. With light weights there is always the temptation to put out the minimum effort needed to move the weight. Allowing yourself to relax when moving a light weight will subvert your heavy training by teaching the body to "turn off" muscles not directly involved.

4. **Kettlebell swing**

    2 sets 10 reps

5. **Kettlebell/Dumbbell Snatch**

    3 sets of 10 reps

6. **Standing dumbbell press**

    3 sets of 5 reps

7. **Overhead Walk**

    2 circuits

8. **Lat Pull Down machine or One arm rowing**

    3 sets of 10 reps

9. **Goblet Squat**

    2 sets of 10 reps

When you finish this session, you should feel strong and like you could do more. What you really want is to be ready for the next round of heavy training. So, enjoy the session and go into your two days of rest primed for heavy lifting.

In conclusion

Planning your training to build toward a personal record attempt in a contest is the best way to insure that you make progress on a regular basis. In this section, I have given you some tools and techniques to do your planning.

Now comes the fun stuff...doing the workouts.

In the next sec   nd deadlift.

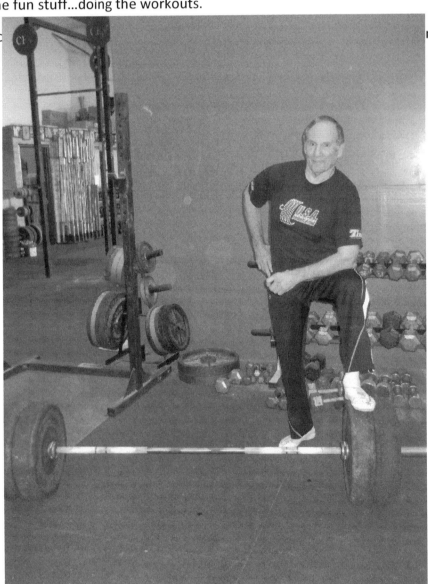

Part II
Training Programs

Food for thought:

"Success in business requires training and discipline and hard work. But if your not frightened by these things, opportunities are just as great today as they ever were."

-David Rockefeller

"Pleasure in the job puts perfection in the work"

-Aristotle

"Work while you have the light. You are responsible for the talent entrusted to you."

Henri Frederic Amiel

PART II

Exercise Programs

The exercise routines that follow are designed to help lifters over age 50 become the strongest they can be. I developed these programs from my own experience, from extensive reading and from some of the great coaching I received over the 25 years I competed.

Most of you are aware that there are an almost endless number of training programs out there. Many lifters search endlessly for "the perfect routine", or the "best combination of sets and reps". They appear to believe that if they could only find the "secret training formula" they would be quickly transformed from mediocre to great.

The real story is perhaps best captured in the expression "the perfect routine is the one you're *not* using". In other words, the idea that there is a perfect routine is pure fantasy.

The programs that follow are all based on the idea that you train **four days a week.** The format is as follows:

> Day 1: Heavy Squat + Assistance work + conditioning work
>
> Day 2: Heavy Bench Press + Assistance work + conditioning work
>
> Day 3: Recovery
>
> Day 4: Heavy Deadlift + Assistance work + conditioning work
>
> Day 5: "Light Day" + conditioning work
>
> Day 6: Recovery
>
> Day 7: Recovery

On each of the heavy lifting days, you will do one of the cycles designed for that lift. It is up to you which you select to do. Each of the cycles will run for 4-8 weeks.

On the "light" lifting day, you will do some very light reps with all three power lifts and do conditioning work.

When you read this, it may seem like a modest work load. Wait until you try it. If you want to get strong, this is an approach that will get you there. When you look at the amount of lifting you do in one week, this is a lot of work.

There may be some people who believe that they need to work out five and six days a week to get better. I have made the point over and over that too much work will make you tired, but not strong.

In the chapters that follow, I'll lay out training cycles for squat, bench press and deadlift. There is no particular need to try to synchronize each lift, other than when you are doing "peaking" training for a contest.

If you have not done powerlifting before, you may want to start out using the basic power

As I have said before and will say again, you need to change your routine every 4-8 weeks to keep getting stronger. That is why training programs for each lift are divided into 4-8 week cycles.

You can re-use these cycles over and over. Just don't repeat the same one you just finished and anticipate progress.

With that general guidance, programs for each of the competition lifts are included in separate chapters. The conditioning routine and the Light Day routine are included after the deadlift chapter.

The big iron awaits you. Go have some fun!

Words of Warning

If you are just beginning powerlifting training, or if you have been doing weight training and performing the power lifts with poor technique, it is imperative that you begin by insuring that your muscles are fully conditioned to do deep squats, bench press with a pause, and deadlifts with correct technique.

You may be particularly at risk if you have not been doing deep squats. Your muscles will be OK with part of the lift, but completely unused to performing when you are in the deep position. This can lead to extreme soreness, cramps or even pulled muscles.

When you begin squatting, you may want to spend two weeks or more getting your body used to the full range of motion in a competition squat. Use very light weights, perhaps beginning with an empty bar. Your body will thank you.

You should also be aware that when you lift heavy weights, you will put your circulatory system under stresses far higher than you may be used to. I strongly suggest you consult with your physician before you begin doing power training.

Chapter 5

The Squat: King of Power Exercises: Proper Technique

The power squat is one of the most demanding lifts in any weight sport. It is athletically and mentally challenging in ways that no other competitive lift is other than the Olympic Snatch and Clean and Jerk.

Squats demand output from every muscle in your body. It is mentally and physically hard to go "below parallel" into a deep squat that is legal for competition.

However, the reward for doing squats is massive body strength. Big squats will even boost your bench press.

Because squats are so technically difficult to do, and because they are one of those athletic activities that feel really hard when you are doing them, most people who lift weights avoid them...or do some lame partial "knee bend".

Now that I have tossed all this macho fertilizer around, let's get down to some useful information.

Later in the next section I'll spend 20+ pages detailing how you do a proper competition squat. There is a lot of detail and all of it is really important. It takes a lot of practice, but stick with it and you will master this very difficult, but rewarding, lift.

Before diving in, let's look at a few of the more common questions people have about doing the squat in weight training.

If you are 50+ years of age, there is a chance that you have some chronic issue with your knees. If you have a question, I would strongly suggest that you get your knees checked out by a sports medicine physician before you try doing squats.

If you do squats using proper technique, they place very limited strain on the knees. If you use bad technique, you will put a *lot* of stress on your knees.

The same goes for your neck and back. Do things right, and no problem at all. Do them wrong, and it is a whole lot of hurt.

Word of warning. Forget everything you have ever learned about doing squats and start from scratch. I would say about 99% of the squats I see in a gym (other than one where powerlifters train) are done with horrible technique.

Most personal trainers have never done a competition squat and have no real idea how to do them. You need to learn how to do it right by carefully following the instructions in the sections that follow.

Technique for Doing a Great Squat

The squat looks deceptively easy. When done perfectly, it looks very easy. It is easy only when you master each part of the lift, and do the *lift exactly the same way each time, regardless of the weight.*

THE Cardinal Rule of Squatting: Stay TIGHT

If you want to build major league strength, you need to pay close attention to critical details that are omitted in most training courses. One of the *critical* things you have to do when building serious power is to *keep all parts of your body under tension, or "tight". This enables you to recruit strength from every part of your body.*

If you are going to put out anything near maximum power, you have to engage every muscle you can to do the lift. You must be certain that you have not "relaxed" some key area of your body, because that will be like having a leak in a hydraulic system. Your lift will collapse into the relaxed area, and your spotters will have to rescue you.

Throughout this book I'll be reminding you to keep all parts of your body tight. This is one of those things that people who have never lifted heavy weights don't understand. Most personal trainers have never lifted a really heavy weight and have no clue what is involved.

If you have not been focusing on getting and staying tight during the squat, you need to start focusing on that the very first day you begin training. This is *absolutely essential* for you to do, otherwise you will be stuck with mediocre results indefinitely.

In this section, I'll cover the basics of what you need to do when building tension in your entire body in order to have a good squat. In sections below, I'll refer to specific things you need to do at various parts of the lift. Make certain you do ALL of them, or you will be struggling with puny weights forever.

Shoulders and upper back

Your shoulders and upper back need to be lock down tight when you pick the weight off the rack. You tense them *before* you lift the weight off the rack, or you won't be able to get them fully engaged.

Your hands should be gripping the bar at a point where your elbows are tight against your body when you take the bar off the rack. *When you grab the bar, you should try to crush it with your grip.* This will activate all the muscles of your arms, upper back and neck.

Your head should be positioned so that you are looking directly ahead of you, or very slightly up. You should *never* arch your head way up like a turtle. You need to keep the same head position throughout the squat. It helps to focus your eyes on a particular point across the room, and keep your gaze there throughout the lift.

Your upper back should be flat, and <u>never</u> "rolled over" or rounded. If it is not flat, you are asking for big trouble in the form of a back injury. You should stand erect, and not bend forward at the waist when the bar in on your back. If any part of your back is rounded, that point is where maximum pressure will be focused when you do your lift. In that case, I hope you have a good hospital nearby.

Core: abdominals and lower back

Your whole back should be flat *with a slight arch in your lower back.* The arch in your lower back will help tighten that area, and also allow you to *flex your abdominal muscles.*

Here is the key to getting your abs tight; you <u>push out</u>. Whatever you do, don't suck your gut in. That will cause your whole core to collapse when you are in the bottom of the squat.

Keeping your core tight involves getting a deep breath that *fills your lower lungs.* This feels like you are filling your belly. Not only will this super deep breath keep your core tight, it will give you much needed oxygen during the lift.

Athletes in many sports from martial arts to competitive running all emphasize the critical importance of "belly breathing". This deep inhalation of air will allow you to have stability in your core when lifting a heavy weight.

Hips, Glutes and Legs

When you have taken the bar off the rack and have stepped back to the position where you are ready to squat, you need to strongly engage the hips and glutes.

Begin by tightening your glutes. The sensation should be that you are squeezing them together. Your hips will kick in when you flex your legs by trying to pull your kneecap up. At the same time, dig your toes into the floor, and try to push your feet apart.

At this point, you are ready to start the squat.

As I'll remind you throughout this book, mastering all of these techniques is difficult. You will have to practice them over and over again. The key thing to remember<u>, the only way you will make progress in lifting is to learn and master better technique.</u> If learning these techniques was easy, everyone would be using them. Most people in gyms will never make any progress beyond the first few months. They will remain novices, and never make progress because they continue to use poor technique.

How to do a Contest Quality Squat

Now I'll break down what you have to do at each stage of the lift. You will be surprised at how many small details must be mastered to do your best at this lift. However, once you use these techniques *every time* you do a squat, the weights you use will increase over time, and you will have the opportunity to realize your own maximum potential.

While it may take less than 30 seconds to actually do a squat, I'm going to take several pages to describe what you should do at each stage of the lift.

The Six Parts of a Squat

To help you learn how to do your best lift, I'll discuss squat technique in six parts.

1. Placing the bar on your back
2. Stepping back from the rack
3. Descending
4. Going below parallel
5. Coming up from the bottom
6. Returning the bar to the rack

In each of these there are a set of things you have to do in order to perform the best, and realize your full potential. It may seem like a lot of detail, but attention to detail is the difference between performing at your full potential, or flopping around like the typical trainee.

Step 1: Placing the Bar on Your Back

Since you will have a lot of weigh on your back, you want to be certain that you don't get into a dangerous situation. I'll cover the ways your set up for lifting can really impact how safe and secure you will be when you squat.

First of all, if possible, squat in a power cage similar to the one in the picture below. The cage has safety bars that can be adjusted in height so that if you can't come up with a squat, you can slowly descend to the height of the safety bars and leave the weight there.

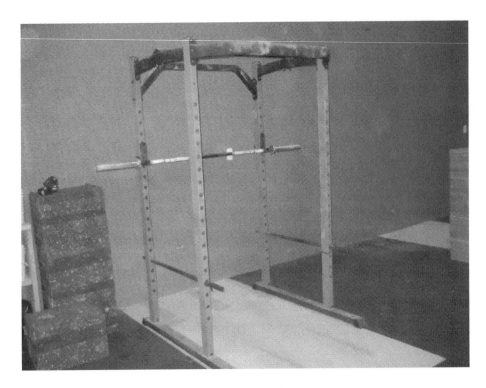

Squat Cage with safety bars

Set the safety bars at a position about 2" below where you will go on the lowest point in your squat. You don't want to hit the bars when you are doing your exercise, but you want them close enough to your bottom point so that you can lower yourself down and release the bar on to them.

There are other squat racks that may have built in safety racks, or have no rack at all. If you use one of these, I recommend that you use a spotter which I'll talk about below.

Step 1A: Set the rack height for your squat bar.

The first thing you do is set the rack height for your squat bar. This is CRITICAL for both performance and for your safety. All squat racks have some way to adjust the height that you place the squat bar so that you can lift it off. *You should select a height where the fully loaded bar will be about the middle of your chest.* This means that you will have to bend your knees to lift the bar off the rack.

<u>*Most important: It means that when you bring the bar back into the rack after doing your lifts, it will be very easy to put back.*</u>   This is a very important issue. You will often see people struggling on their tip toes to put a squat bar back in the rack. This is what we call "being in Death Valley". One small slip and you have a huge accident.

For your own safety, and the safety of people around you, it is critical that you be able to walk forward and <u>lower</u> the bar onto the rack.

Making it easy to replace the bar after a heavy squat is really important for your safety. You cannot imagine how badly you could be injured if you had to *raise* the bar on tip toes, putting each end back on the rack separately…and one end missed the rack. The end where you missed the rack would instantly drop, and depending on the weight could really do major damage to your back, arms, neck, etc. Look at the picture for an example of how to set your rack height.

So….for your own safety, set the rack at a height where you can simply walk straight ahead and *lower* the squat bar back into the rack.

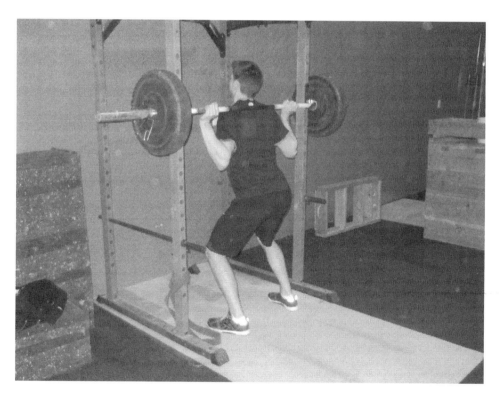

Proper rack height for this lifter to take the bar off the rack

Step 1B: Placing the squat bar on your back.

<u>This may be the single most important part of this book</u>, so read the following section carefully and practice it until you have mastered it. If you don't place the bar on your back properly, all the other advice in this program is of minimal value.

<u>Got your attention?</u>

Remember what I told you that it was necessary to master all the little details for you to reach your full potential. I am going to teach you a version of the squat that will be perfect for your conditioning, but will use the technique used by serious power athletes.

The first thing you do is set your grip set on the bar so that when you put the bar on your back, you will be in the exact center of the bar. If you are positioned even an inch one way or the other, a heavy weight may seem seriously out of balance when you take it off the rack.

Every workout bar has ring markings at even intervals. Use these markings to insure that you set your grip *at exactly the same spot on each side of the bar.*

Most people prefer to place their hands so that they have between 6 and 12 inches from their shoulder to their hand. The pictures below will show lifters with slightly different grip placement. The thing that is uniform for all of them is that every grip keeps the lifter in the center of the bar, and allows them to get tight.

One thing to consider is that you don't want to run the risk of pinching your hand when you set the bar back on the rack. For people under 6' 2" this is generally not a problem. Larger individuals may want to have a wider grip on the squat bar, and then have to make certain that they don't pinch their hands (or worse) when they set the bar back on the rack.

People who need to grip the bar all the way out to the collars may opt to use squat racks that can be set closer together so that they can safely grip the bar at the collar. If you chose this option, it is always best to use spotters on all your lifts.

One additional note on the way you grip the bar. *You must always grip the bar with all your fingers, and must try to crush the bar with your grip when you squat.* It may sound odd to some of you, but if you have a relaxed grip on the bar, you will be relaxed in your arms and shoulders. This translates to putting out far less force than you could. I will stress over and over then absolute necessity of recruiting power from every part of your body when you do a big lift. If any part of you is relaxed, you will do a sub-optimal lift.

Now that you have your grip on the bar, it is time to put it on your back.

Place the bar across the back of your shoulders about 2 to 3 inches below your neck. *Do not place the bar way up on your neck or your trapezius muscles.* Look at the photograph and see where the bar is placed. Placing the bar here will insure that you are supporting the load with across the widest and strongest part of your upper body. If you have the bar "high" up on your neck, you will be trying to lift a huge load supported by a narrow and very vulnerable part of your body. You can feel the vertebra in your neck. There is NO muscle between them and the surface of your skin. You REALLY DON'T want to put a heavy metal bar against the exposed vertebra of you neck.

How much difference can bar placement make in your ability to support and control weight? I'm 5'10" tall and weigh 180 pounds. The most I can take off the rack with the bar positioned up on my neck is about 225 lbs. When I'm doing heavy training for competition squatting, with the bar placed across my shoulders, I will routinely lift 600-700 pounds a few inches to build my spinal erectors. My best full squat in competition in the past five years has been 436.

So you see….the impact of bar placement is HUGE!

When you are lifting, your elbows should be under the bar. By driving them forward you lock the bar into position on your back. Driving them forward also keeps your chest up and your back tensed and flat. These are necessities for moving any serious iron.

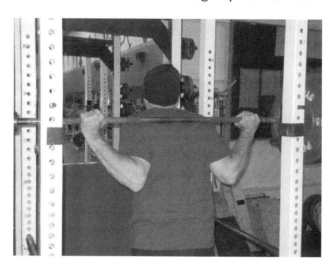

Correct placement for the bar in a squat

If you have been training with the bar placed up on your neck, it may take a while to get used to the feel of having it placed lower. Work with light weights and find the positioning that is best for you. When things are "right" the bar should feel very stable on your back. It will feel like the bar is "locked" onto your back and you have complete control of the bar and the weight during your lift.

<u>WARNING: Do NOT</u> use a pad or a towel wrapped around the bar. The only reason pads are ever used in squatting is because the bar is placed too high…basically up on the *neck.* You are placing a heavy weight on the most vulnerable part of your body. Most personal trainers teach the squat this way because *they* have never lifted heavy weights. If you want a sore neck (or worse), and guarantee that you make little or no progress, do the squat with the bar on your neck.

One caveat is appropriate here. Olympic style lifters use a version of the squat that is called the "high bar" squat. Generally, they will not be squatting with much more than they can put overhead. I trained this way when I did Olympic lifting, and it is a technique often taught in Cross Fit gyms. Unless you are training specifically for Olympic lifting, I strongly recommend that you *not* use the high bar technique. The main reason is that you will reach your maximum lift at a *much lower* weight than by using the technique I describe in this program.

Step 2: Stepping Back from the Rack

Once you have the bar placed securely on your back, you are ready to remove it from the rack and set up to do a squat. There are a few important things to do during this phase of the lift.

Step 2A: Standing up under the bar.

Taking a weighted bar off a rack is easy when the weight is light, but becomes very tricky when the weight gets heavy. For that reason, you should do each move in a manner that gives you maximum stability and control.

Begin by settling under the bar while it is still on the rack. You adjust yourself so that you are positioned with the bar resting exactly where it will be when you lift it off. When you are in position, you tense every muscle in your body. You should crush the bar with your grip. Take a deep breath and hold it. You are now ready to lift the bar off the rack.

It is extremely important that your back be flat, and not rounded at any point. You are going to lift a big weight off a rack, and it is critical that your spine be in the best position to support the weight.

You should stand erect, with your feet spaced just about under your shoulders. Pause briefly to see if the bar is evenly loaded on your back. If it is not, immediately replace the bar in the rack. Don't ever try to lift a bar that is unevenly loaded. See the picture for correct lift off position.

Keeping your body tight throughout this lift is critical. If any muscle group relaxes, it is like having a leak in a hydraulic system. Everything collapses toward the leak.

If everything is loaded properly, and you feel ready, it is time to step back to the position where you will do the squat.

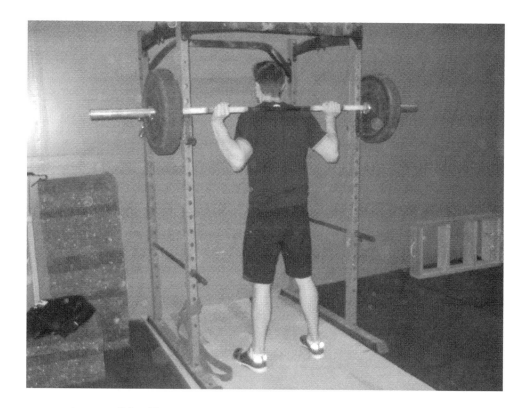

Correct lift off position – ready to step back to perform squat

Step 2B: Stepping back into squatting position

The key to success here is to use the <u>minimum number of steps to get into position to begin the squat.</u> If you have watched inexperienced (and some experienced) lifters squat, you will notice that they will often take several small steps to get into position where they feel ready to squat. *Any extra steps you take with a big weight on your back will drain your strength you want to use for squatting!*

One key to success is minimizing the steps you take on the "walk out" and being ready to begin your descent as quickly as possible.

You can practice your "walk out" with an empty bar across your back. By doing this you can learn quickly how to get into position with two to four steps, rather than wandering all over.

Your goal is to wind up in the position to begin the descent with the weight stable on your back.

Step 2C: Foot Spacing

All good squatters prefer a foot spacing that is wider than their shoulders. The object is to find a foot spacing that will enable you to use the biggest muscles in your body (gluteus and hamstrings) at critical points of the lift. Each person has slightly different leverages, so you will need to experiment to see which works best for you. The picture below shows an initial optimal foot spacing.

Over time you should move your feet out a few more inches. This really helps engage the glutes and hamstrings in the low part of the lift. Ultimately you want to develop a relatively wide stance to fully engage the glutes and hamstrings in the bottom of the lift.

You should never take a "narrow" stance, as the only muscles engaged in the lift are the quads on the front of your legs. They need help from the glutes and the hamstrings if you are going to lift some big iron.

Some lifters who use supportive squat suits will take a *very* wide stance. That really only works if you are wearing one of the specialized powerlifting support suits. This program is aimed at the vast majority of lifters and athletes who lift without support gear.

When your feet are in position, you will probably want to take two or three deep breaths before beginning the squat. Hold the last breath from the just before beginning the descent until you are almost back to an upright standing position. You *must hold your breath during the descent and ascent part of the squat.* If you release the breath it means you will relax....and the weight will suddenly seem to become much heavier.

Stand erect with your knees straight and your chest up. Your back should be straight with no rounding anywhere. The weigh should be solid on your back.

The picture below shows the position you should be in when ready to begin your descent.

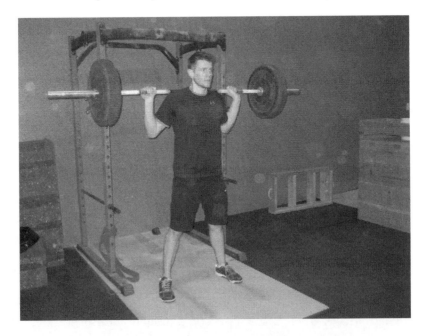

Ready to begin descent. Note foot position.

Once you have your feet in position, you should tense up all the muscles that will support you during the squat. Dig your toes into the floor, tighten your calves, push out with your feet, and tighten your abdominal muscles by pushing them out. Your whole body should be tight and ready to put out full power.

Keep your head erect, and look at a something directly in front of you. If you are looking at a wall, pick a spot on the wall and keep your eyes there for the entire lift. If you are looking out into a room, pick a spot near the back of the room and keep your eyes focused on that during the entire lift.

You should practice staying tight during the entire lift. This is one of those things you can do that will train your neuromuscular system to work at full power. The key is insuring that you always stay tight regardless of the weight on your back.

Step 3: The Descent

Breathing: Proper breathing in the squat is absolutely critical if you are going to do your best. Breathing is part of staying tight and insuring you have good mechanics when doing the lift.

When you are standing erect ready to begin descending, take at least one _deep_ breath, _and then hold it throughout the squat until you have come all the way back up._

A serious athletic deep breath means that you fill _all of your lungs._ Most people fill only the top part of their lungs. You should drive breath deep into your abdomen. This practice of "belly breathing" discussed earlier is absolutely critical to keeping you tight and putting out full power.

When you take a deep breath and holding it, you accomplish two things. One is to provide the oxygen your body will need for doing a heavy lift. The second is that by holding the deep breath you create an inflated "balloon" that will compress when you are in the bottom of the squat. Your inflated lungs will literally help you get a drive out of the deepest part of the squat.

One of the things you should consciously avoid is taking several _shallow_ breaths. Inexperienced lifters will often take a lot of shallow breaths, and in the process spend a lot of extra time with a big weight on your back. Shallow breathing also never fills up your lower lungs.

It may be useful for you to practice doing the walk out to the starting position and then taking a proper deep breath. You can do this with a light weight.

The descent – Proper Mechanics: You begin the descent with your chest held up. You should keep your *chest up throughout the lift*. This will keep your back flat, and keep the bar positioned where you have the most control over it.

The first movement downward should be "sitting back" as if you were going to sit in a chair. The most powerful squat movement will be one where you keep your shins nearly straight up and down.

You should keep your eyes focused on a spot in the room that is roughly the same level as your head. Keeping your chest up and your shoulders rolled slightly back. This will keep your body alignment correct.

You should try to keep your shins straight up and down. Generally, your knees will drift forward a bit, but you should *never* allow your knees to go ahead of a line rising vertically from your toes. When you do this, you do this you put a huge strain on the knees. It also means the weight is now moving forward, and you are in danger of going nose down and ass up with the barbell on your back.

If you train regularly in a gym where there are few people doing heavy squats, you are probably exposed to some pretty dreadful squatting technique. You should really try not to watch it, and focus only on developing your own perfect form.

Now, here is where the Russians have come up with an idea that is almost foolproof for developing good squatting technique. The cool thing about this is that the drill is nearly painless, and can be done without any weight. If you perform this drill, you will virtually insure that you can develop perfect squatting technique.

This drill is called "The Wall Squat". Don't confuse this version with the exercise where you hold your back against the wall in a squat position and do an isometric hold. This is the version where you *face* the wall, and teach your body how to be perfectly aligned to do a barbell squat.

Begin by facing the wall, with your feet in squatting position (wider than shoulder width), and your toes *touching* the wall. Hold your hands down in front of you. Your face will be against the wall. Now, descend to a point where your thighs are parallel to the floor. Then descend into a position where you are "below parallel".

The first time they try the wall squat, most people will fall over backwards, or lose their balance. Don't worry about that. Keep working on the drill until you can easily do five reps with proper form to full depth. This is the exact technique you should use *to do barbell squats*.

One of the first things you will discover is that you have to spread your knees as you descend. This is what you should be doing, since it is going to activate the big muscles in your glutes and hamstrings for a push out of the bottom.   You will also find that you have to keep your shins almost vertical do a proper descent. This again is good technique.

Working against the wall you *have* to keep your head up, chest up, and your back flat. Rather than roll your knees forward to do a squat, you stick your rear end back like you were sitting down. Again….this is exactly what you should be doing. I don't know of a better or easier way for someone to learn how to squat properly.

Use this exact same form when you do the barbell squat, and you will develop a lot of body strength with little risk of injury.   Be diligent about using proper form and you will master the technique needed to do superior lifts.

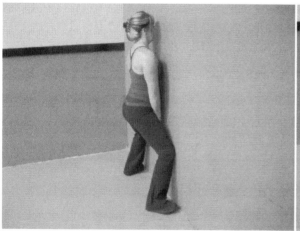 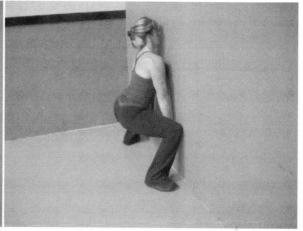

Starting Position for Wall Squat   **Descent: the wall forces you to have perfect form - Go all the way down!**

It is easier to learn to do something right the first time than to spend the rest of your life trying to correct your mistakes.

It will help you to practice the wall squat regularly, even when you have been squatting for decades. It helps keep your technique in good order. It is really difficult to achieve consistency with any complex movement. The squat is a very technically complex athletic movement. All competitive lifters regularly work on perfecting their technique. When you practice form, you are doing what the "big dogs" do.

Step 4: Going Below Parallel

Getting below parallel is one of the tougher things in weigh sports. "The Hole" as it is known is one of the scarier places for any lifter, especially with a big load on their back.   It is also where real strength is built, along with flexibility and athleticism.

You have the best chance to consistently go below parallel if you keep your chest up during the descent, and keep your hips low. Many times people will begin to bend forward at the waist when they near parallel, and when this happens, it becomes very difficult to get below parallel.

By keeping your chest up, and "sitting" down into the squat, you have the best chance to consistently break the parallel plain. You can get the feel of this by consistently practicing the "wall squat" described above.

When you are at the deepest point in the squat, your body is under the most pressure from the weigh and from being compressed. It is absolutely essential that you not let any breath escape, or relax any muscles. If you lose tension it will be very difficult (perhaps impossible) to return to the standing position.

To insure that you are consistently able to get below parallel, it is good practice to have one or two training partners watch your lifts. They should watch you from the side, with their eyes at the level of your hip. No one can tell anything if they are standing behind you, and their view is distorted if they are standing with their eyes above (or below) your hip level. The picture shows a legitimate "deep" squat.

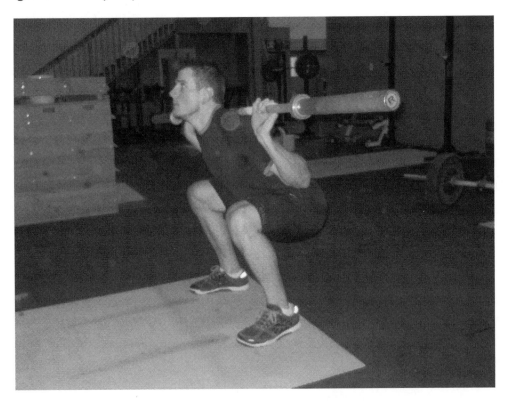

Below Parallel – Top of knee is above the top of the thigh

These people should tell you the truth, even if it hurts. All too often friends tell us what they think we want to hear. The people who critique your lifts should give you real feedback, and then you can do what is necessary to correct any problems.

Once you are below parallel, it is time to hit the thrust reversers and stand up with the weight on your back.

Step 5: Coming out of the Bottom

If there are two words that describe what you must do to come out of the bottom of a big squat they are: EXPLODE and SPEED!

In any move that develops real power, it is *absolutely essential that you move the weight as <u>fast</u> as you can. If you are not moving the weight as fast as you can, you are NOT putting out maximum power.*

Lifters who move the weight at a slow speed are putting out anywhere from 40% to maybe 70% of their actual capacity.

Focus every single bit of tension you can muster to blast out of the bottom as quickly as you can.

Having said that….it is important that your *lifting technique* be as close to perfect as possible to take full advantage of your power output. When you "explode", it is *absolutely essential* that you not relax any part of your body or lose your form. You have to drive the bar upward with a very tight and precisely aligned body.

Assuming that your foot spacing is wider than your shoulders, you will have set up properly for two of the biggest muscles in your body to engage when you are deep in the hole (glutes and hamstrings). If your foot spacing is too narrow, you will throw almost all the work onto the quads, and you will have a very difficult time getting out of the bottom of the squat.

When you begin to come up, your chest should move up first. Many lifters have the bad habit of moving their hips upward to begin recovering from a deep squat. What this does is suddenly throw the primary stress of lifting the weigh onto your lower back. It also means you can become bent way forward, which is a very high risk position to be in with a heavy weight on your back.

Keeping the chest high during the drive out of the bottom of the lift is essential. This keeps the weight positioned over your hips and means that you are getting the most efficient push from your legs and back. This position is not only the most efficient for pushing up out of the bottom, it also allows you to keep control of the weight far better than if you start to assume a "bent over" posture.

If you feel like you are starting to "bend over", one thing you can do is to consciously push your elbows forward and up. This will elevate your chest, and help restore the alignment you want. At the same time, drive your hips forward. This will keep you in the optimal chest up position.

Using the "wall squat" shown above to practice the explosion out of the bottom can be very helpful.

Another thing the wall squat will show you is that your knees should be spread rather than collapsing inward. If your knees begin to sag inward at any time during the upward part of the lift, you should consciously push them out. This keeps you exerting maximum power for the upward push.

Just above the point where your thighs are parallel to the floor is the dreaded "sticking point". This is where the drive upward can stall because you are shifting the main load of moving the weight from your glutes and hamstrings to your quads. You can get a nice drive out of the bottom, but suddenly stall out at the "sticking point".

What you want to do is literally blast past the sticking point and use your upward momentum to keep you driving toward standing erect with a big weight. Getting past the sticking point is another reason to move the weight as fast as you can during the ascent.

The quads are the primary driver for the final portion of the lift. Once past the sticking point, you will continue your push until you are at the lock out position, standing erect.

You are just about to finish the lift. But there are a few more things to be aware of.

First of all, you want to reach the top of the lift smoothly and not have the bar bounce on your shoulders. You have been driving upward as fast as you can, but as you near the top, it is essential that you slow down for a smooth arrival. The last thing you want is for the bar to keep on going upward, and fall back down on your shoulders.

Think of your deceleration at the top of the lift much like an elevator in a very tall building. The car goes very fast from floor 5-70, but slows down for a smooth arrival at floor 75.

Finally, it is really important to finish the lift with your knees straight not bent. However, you should *never lock your knees,* especially with a heavy weight on your back. Locking the knees in any athletic movement is a dangerous and potentially crippling move. Finish with your knees straight....but not locked.

Step 6: Returning the Bar to the Rack

When you have stood upright with the squat bar, there are a few things to do to complete the lift safely.

First, be certain the bar is steady on your back before stepping toward the rack. If you are unstable for any reason, you can get in trouble quickly once you start walking with the weight on your back.

Second, don't relax until you have put the weight on the rack. You have to stay tight to control the bar, so wait until it is firmly on the rack before you relax.

Third, walk the bar back into the rack. If you have positioned the rack properly, all you will have to do is walk straight in, allow the bar to hit the uprights, and then allow the weigh to drop *down* onto the rack. If you have to work *to raise* the bar to get it back on the rack, you have set the rack too high.

I can't stress how important it is to have the rack set at a height that allows you to walk straight in and allow the bar to settle *down* onto the rack. If you are handling a heavy weight the *last* thing you want to do is try to *raise* a heavy bar to try to get it back on the rack. That will eventually lead to a bad accident where you completely lose control of the weight.

Spotting the Squat

If you are going to do heavy squats, your personal safety should be a paramount concern. This is one lift where you can get in trouble quickly, and need to have a way to safely get out from under the loaded bar.

If there is one thing that anyone intending to do big squats should know, it is how to spot properly. If you are the lifter, you need to insure that your spotters know what to do. If you are spotting, it is essential that you know how to do it properly. Inept spotters can cause serious injury to a lifter. Perhaps more surprising is that if the spotters don't know what they are doing, *they* can be badly injured.

You should know how to *instruct* people to spot you when you lift, and know how to do spotting for others. This may save you or someone else a great deal of pain.

You should always use one spotter standing behind you. If you have a very heavy weight you can add spotters on each end. Regardless, the spotter standing behind you will do the same things.

One spotter Technique – When using a single spotter, the person spotting positions themselves just behind the lifter. The spotter will keep their hands under the lifters arms with palms open so if needed that they can apply force to the lifters rib cage. Look at the picture to see proper positioning of the hands.

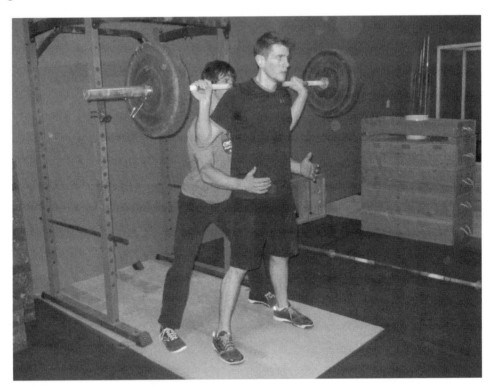

Beginning position for spotting the squat

The spotter should NOT touch the lifter unless the lifter asks for help! The spotter is in position to help if needed, but any touching of the lifter will create a major distraction. In competitive lifting events, if the spotter touches the lifter in any way, the lift is considered no good.

The lifter and the spotter should agree before the lift begins as to how the lifter will ask for help. When both spotter and lifter understand what signal will be used, the lift can begin.

The spotter should be ready to help from the first. The lifter may have trouble lifting the bar off the rack, and need help putting it back. In order to help, the spotter should be positioned 12 to 18 inches behind the lifter during the entire lift.

Once the lifter is in position, standing erect ready to start the squat, the spotter should have their hands positioned so that they can apply pressure to the lifters rib cage area. The spotter will be reaching around the lifters torso, but *never actually touching the lifter unless* <u>*the lifter asks for help.*</u>

As the lifter descends, the spotter will have keep their hands a few inches below the lifters rib cage. In other words, the spotter will "follow" the lifters movement down and up.

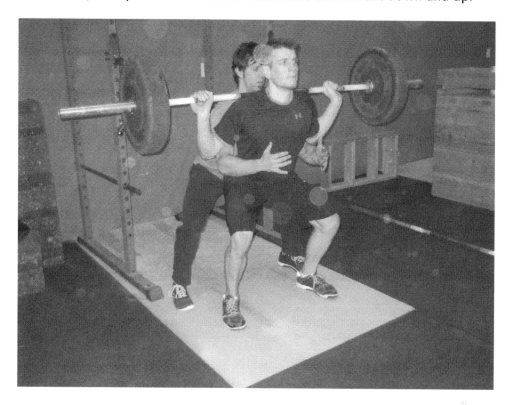

Correct position for spotting the squat

If the lifter asks for help, the spotter should immediately do the following:

1. Place both hands on the lifters lower rib cage, and <u>*stabilize the lift.*</u> The first thing that needs to be done is to prevent the lifter from getting in any more difficulty.
2. Once stabilized, the spotter can apply modest pressure to the rib cage area and in tandem with the lifter, return to the starting position, and place the bar back on the rack. The spotter needs to only apply 20-30 pounds of pressure to the lifter, enough to get them moving again.

It is essential that in recovering from a failed squat attempt, the lifter and the spotter work together to get the bar back up to the squat rack. The lifter <u>*must never abandon the bar, or quit trying to get it back to the rack.*</u>   The spotter can stabilize the bar, and help the lifter get it back in the rack. It is not the spotter's job to take the entire weight off the lifter.

If you are lifting in a squat cage, the spotter can assist the lifter in lowering the bar to the safety bars. When the bar is on the safety bars, the lifter can crawl out from under the weight now resting on the bars.

One serious word of warning…

NEVER EVER simply "dump" the bar off your back and let it fall behind you. This is very very dangerous for the lifter, and extremely dangerous to any spotter standing behind you.

Unfortunately, some lifters who use rubberized plates will dump a weight regularly in their training. When you drop a barbell behind you the chance that it will hit your lower back is pretty high. The consequences of being hit by a barbell loaded for even a "light" squat can be catastrophic.

One of the greatest women powerlifters of all time was injured in an accident where she dropped the bar behind her. At the peak of her career, she was able to squat over 600 lbs in competition. In the decade since her accident, she can no longer lift weights, has endured many surgeries, has done countless hours of rehabilitation, and has to walk with a cane for the rest of her life. In short, "dumping" the bar turned her from a great athlete to someone who can't walk normally and is in constant pain.

Moral of the story: always use a spotter if there is a chance you will need assistance.

Using spotters on each end of the bar. If you are lifting a very heavy weight, it is sensible to have additional spotters on each end of the bar. The job of these spotters is to assist the spotter standing behind the lifter in the event that the lifter gets in trouble.

The most important thing for spotters on the ends of the bar to remember is *stabilize the bar if the lifter gets in trouble.* <u>Do NOT pull the bar upward until all three spotters AND the lifter, are ready to move the bar upward.</u>

If one of the spotters on the end of the bar suddenly pulls upward, it can throw the lifter completely off balance, and tilt the majority of the weight over on to the opposite spotter. This can result in the lifter being injured, and the other spotters being put at high risk.

Chapter 6

Power Training Cycles for Squats

Building major body power with squats requires that you are mentally and physically committed to working hard, and keeping your focus. Serious power training is not simply breezing through a few sets of an exercise. It involves mastering intense mental focus, training your body to give maximum output for a few seconds, routinely doing a wide range of small movements correctly every time, and discovering how to enjoy this process.

By now you have probably figured out that if someone can write well over 10 pages on how to do one exercise movement, there must be a lot of small details that need attention. That's true.

What is not immediately obvious to some is that the fact that you are fit and strong enough to take on this challenge is a true blessing. Few people are actually able to do the workouts described below, and if you are one of the fortunate ones, you should feel grateful.

In that spirit, I'll describe a series of exercise programs that will help you build massive body power using the squat as a critical tool.

Many people try to become strong, but few actually realize even half their potential. Generally, this is because those who fall short don't utilize their mind as well as their body in the quest for super strength. In the workouts that follow, you will have to actually *learn and apply* some things that may be new to you. If you devote the energy, focus and effort needed, you will be rewarded with strength far beyond what you believed was possible.

The thing that will distinguish the super achiever from the person who just gets average results will be how diligently they are willing to practice all the small things that go into creating a big lift. The key to success is in mastering the details.

Warm Up for Squatting

Your power training workout begins as soon as you start to warm up. The warm up is an integral part of your training, and should be given careful attention. Most people just slop around. You need to be focused and treat the warm up as a very important part of your "practice" to lift big iron.

Your objective in the warm up is to get ready to put our maximum force. However, you should *train* your body to be ready to lift heavy with a *minimum* of energy expenditure. This is a trick from the martial arts. Get ready quickly for maximum effort.

When most people think of a "warm up", they think of doing many sets and many reps. For example, at powerlifting meets I often see competitors do a huge number of squats during their warm ups. They start with a set of 10 at 135 and then increase the weight and do more sets of 5, 3 and so forth. Eventually, they have done anywhere from 15 to 25 squats to 'warm up' for their first attempt.

I have trained myself so that most often I'll do a single (perfect) rep at 135, another perfect rep at 225 and finally at a weight about 50 pounds below my opening attempt. In short, my "warm up" is a total of 3 squats. My body is just as ready to lift as anyone who has done 25 squats (or more).

The big difference is that I have expended far less energy doing 3 squats in my warm up than the person who has done 25 squats. I put that energy into the heavy squats.

A warm up for heavy lifting is activating not only the muscles, but also your central nervous system that will control how much force you can apply. You do this by being conscious that you need to prepare both of these systems to function effectively with a very few practice repetitions.

The way you learn to do this rapid warm up is *mental focus.* You train your mind to command your body to be "ready" in absolute minimum time. You mentally visualize yourself doing a heavy squat. At that time, you literally "feel" yourself being ready for full power output.

Visualization is one of the greatest performance enhancers ever developed. It is used by elite athletes in all sports. It a subject covered in many other publications. You can begin to learn this powerful technique by practicing it in your warm up routine.

Here is a warm up routine that you can use to get ready for a very productive squat training session. Remember, the warm up is a critical part of your preparation to do a maximum lift and you should treat it as an integral part of your training.

Jack knife movement – This is movement that strengthens the core area, and loosens the muscles of the lower back and hips. You begin in push up position, with hands immediately below the shoulders, and balanced on your toes with feet spread about 18 inches apart.

Begin by pushing your rear end into the air while keeping the arms straight. Then you drop the hips and bend at the waist keeping your chest up. Your arms are straight and you are still supported on your hands and toes. (see photos)

This may be a challenging move at first. You will gradually get much stronger and more flexible. Begin by doing about 10-15 reps of this movement. Eventually work up to the point where you are doing one rep for each year of your age.

This movement may not look "cool", and the odds are that no one else in the gym does it. However, it will build up core strength and flexibility in ways that almost no other movement will. You will also get your shoulders ready for supporting some big iron.

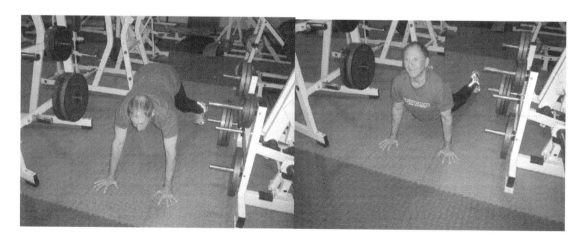

Jack Knife – Start Position　　　　　　　　**Jack Knife – Finish position**

Unweighted Squat – This will help you insure that you are ready to go through the full range of motion of the squat. Simply fold your arms across your chest and lower yourself as far down as you can go in the squat position. If you are stiff, take a few reps to get down to rock bottom.

Do a total of 10 unweighted squats to insure you are ready to lift through the whole range of the squat motion.

Wall Squat – The wall squat shown earlier in this book should be done to get your body ready to do a proper squat to proper depth. You should do a minimum of five wall squats. When you are finished you know that your body is "dialed in" on doing a perfect squat.

Barbell Squat - At this point do **2** sets of the barbell squat with super light weights. Begin with a minimal weight and do the first rep perfectly. You can do 2 or 3 more reps if you need to.

Eventually, you want to do no more than a total of 2 squats before you begin your training session.

Remember, you are aiming at doing every rep perfectly every time. NEVER listen to the yahoo's who say "I can't get deep until the weight is heavy". The chances are that these types will never go deep on a heavy squat….they have programmed themselves to fail.

Now let's check out the squat training cycles.

Squat Cycle #1 - The Foundation Program (aka. 5 x 5 Program)

The "5 by 5" approach is one of the most widely used strength building approaches in weight training. If you are new to squatting or have not been squatting for a while, this is a great program that will get you into condition to move some serious iron.

If you do powerlifting for many years, you will revisit this program frequently.

This program is 5 sets of 5 reps, all done at a percentage of your best 1 rep maximum squat at the beginning of the program. If you have done a recent 1 rep max lift, you can use that. If you have not squatted heavy for a while, see the section on estimating your 1 rep max lift.

As a general rule, it is *much* better to begin with a low estimate. You will make progress rapidly as the weeks go by. If you start too high, you will plateau quickly.

You should do this work out **once a week**, for **8 weeks.** At the end of eight weeks you will begin a new training routine. If 5 sets is too many for you to do and recover, eliminate the last set.

You are now ready to squat. *Review all the earlier materials on how to do the squat properly. You should do every set and every rep with perfect form.*

You will be doing 5 sets of 5 reps each set. Each set will be a percentage of your current maximum squat.

    Set 1 = 50% of 1 rep maximum

    Set 2 = 70% of 1 rep max

    Set 3 = 80% of 1 rep max

    Set 4 = 70% of 1 rep max

    Set 5 = 60% of 1 rep max

Depending on how difficult the set is, take anywhere from 2-5 minutes to recover between sets. Since you are building strength, you need to be well recovered before you begin the next set.

If you did every squat to proper depth, you will have really done what you need to do to build great power.

Increasing the weight: Increase the weight each <u>week</u>, not every workout.

If you calculated your 1 rep max properly, you should be able to add about 5 pounds to the 80% set each week. Over 8 weeks that will be an increase of 40 pounds. You should also be able to add 5 pounds to your 70% sets.

If you can't continually add weight, it is OK to stay at a weight for a couple weeks. What you don't want to do is start with too heavy a weight and not be able to make increases regularly. Starting too close to your limit will mean your progress quickly stalls, and may actually go in reverse.

When you have finished your squats, you go to your assistance exercises. These are designed to build muscle that will support development of a big league squat.

Most of your energy will go into the 5 x 5 squat sets you do. The assistance work in this program will be done to help build up your muscles that support the squat.

Assistance Exercises

Kettlebell Swing – This exercise is one that when done correctly will really build up your posterior power chain. If you don't have kettlebells handy, you can use a dumbbell, and grip one end.

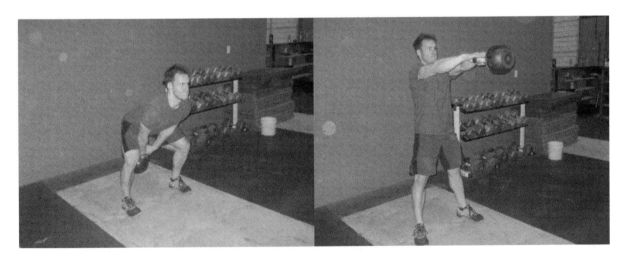

Swing – starting position   **Swing – top position**

In the swing I recommend, the weight will never travel higher than a position where your arms are parallel to the floor.

You begin by swinging the weight back between your legs as if you were hiking a football. Keep your back flat, chest up and eyes straight ahead. Keep your eyes on a spot on the wall at just above eye level for the entire exercise. When the weight has swung back, drive it forward and up by quickly straightening your legs. At the same time, stand upright.

The weight should be propelled upward by your legs and your abdominal muscles. Your arms are nothing but the "ropes" used to connect the weight to your body. You should feel the exercise in your abdominal muscles, in your glutes and the hamstrings. If you feel it in your lower back, your posture is "rolled over" and you are not doing the movement correctly.

You should begin using a moderately heavy dumbbell or kettlebell (kettlebell preferred) and start doing 2 sets of 10-15 reps. You should work up to doing 2 sets of 25 reps with the same moderately heavy weight.

This movement will build great power in your core area.

Back Hyperextension

Building the strength of your hamstrings and glutes is critical to building a powerful athletic body. The back hyperextension does a great job of building both strength and muscular endurance.

If you have not done this exercise before, begin without holding any extra weights. You need to get your hamstrings and glutes used to working through the full range of motion in this lift before stressing them to the max. Begin by doing **2 sets of 10 reps** without any extra weight. Work up to doing **2 sets of 25 reps** without weight before you start holding barbell plates against your chest.

Once you are conditioned to do 25 reps in this movement, you can try holding a barbell plate against your chest and doing **10 reps.** Once you begin holding barbell plates, keep the repetitions at 10, and add weight to the exercise once per week.

It is important that you do the hyperextension through the full range of motion. You need to lower your trunk so that at the bottom of the movement, you are at a 90-degree angle with the floor. At the top, raise your trunk so that your trunk is above a parallel position to the floor. See the pictures for proper position.

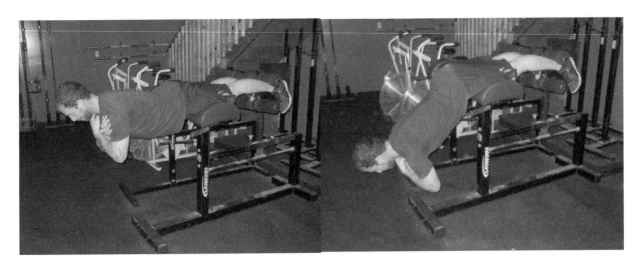

Back Hyperextension – Top Position   **Back Hyperextension – Lower Position**

Hanging Leg Raise

Building strong abs is critical if you are going to have a good squat. The hanging leg raise is one of those movements that will pay huge dividends if your practice it regularly.

You begin by hanging from a chin up bar with your legs straight down. You should not hang limply from the bar, but should have a tight grip with your hands, and pull your body slightly up with your lats and shoulders. To recruit a lot of power to this movement, your upper body needs to have tension throughout the lift.

There are two versions of this lift. Depending on your current conditioning, you may be able to do the exercise with your legs straight. Most people will need to begin with the version where you raise the knees up rather than raise a straight leg.

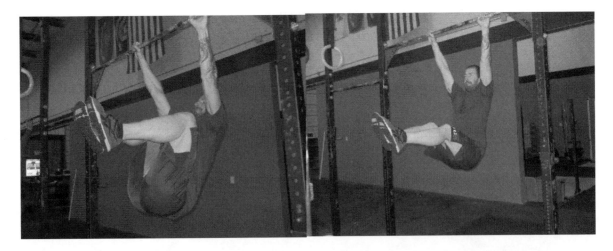

Hanging Leg Raise – Knees to Chest   **Hanging Leg Raise – Legs Extended**

You will be raising the knees to a position where the top of your thigh has gone above parallel with the floor. Begin by doing **2 sets of 10 reps.** Add repetitions until you can do **2 sets of 20 reps.**

At that point, switch to the version of the exercise where you raise a straight leg to a position that is above parallel to the floor. Rather than do a set number of sets and reps, begin by doing as many sets as you need to get **10 total reps.** Work up until you can do **20 total reps.**

That is plenty of work for one training session.

It is important not to over work during this training routine. You should leave the gym feeling like you could "do some more". If you fall victim to the temptation to train to near exhaustion each session, you will quickly stop making progress. Your body will not be able to recover and build strength between training sessions.

One more point that is really important if you want to build strength; training "to failure" is a clear pathway to failure. If you recall the earlier discussion about teaching your body to put out full power for a single rep, you will recall that the higher the number of reps, the less actual power you are putting into any one rep. Training to failure basically insures that you never learn how to put out maximum force.

Remember this Success Tip: *Keep a written record of every set, rep and weight for the entire eight-week cycle. That way you can track your progress, and see what is working best for you.*

At the end of the eight-week cycle, try for a new current 1 rep max lift.

On the first workout day of the week after you have finished the 8-week cycle, warm up properly, and see what you can do now for a 1 rep maximum squat. You should use spotters on all your heavy lifts, so be certain to get someone to help you who knows what they are doing.

Squat Cycle #2 - Partial Squats and Deep Pause Squats

In the second squat program, I'll introduce you to using static contraction training along with "speed" squats. This is a program you will stay on for **4 weeks** before you change to another.

Static contraction training involves doing partial repetitions with weights that are much heavier than you could use doing a full squat. You are training your muscles to handle a much heavier load than you would use for a personal record attempt. The benefit of this is that when you do a heavy single rep, it will feel lighter on your back than it would otherwise.

You are also going to train your muscles to put out full power with some "speed work".

It is critical that you maintain proper squat form for all of the movements in this training program. There is always a temptation to alter you form when doing partial movements, or movements with light weights. You should be very careful to insure that when you do the two lifts below you insure that your body position is in the exact alignment that it would be when you were doing a full squat.

Partial Squats –

This will introduce you to the "power cage" and a few of the many ways you can use this to train.

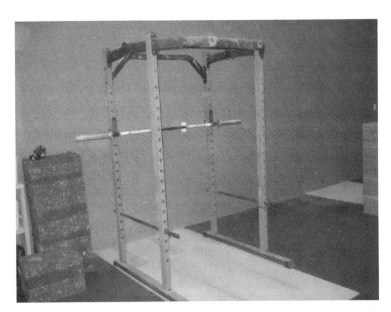

You will note that the power cage has metal safety bars that can be adjusted to different heights. This feature will allow you to handle weights that are much heavier than you would be able to manage ordinarily.

This program will introduce you to one of the uses of the power cage, partial squats.

This exercise should be done **inside** a power cage with safety bars. The bars should be set at a height that will allow you to set the weight down if you can't do the movement. The power cage is one of the greatest training tools you can ever use to build great strength and power.

You will do partial squats with the safety bars set at **2 different heights.** In the exercise, you will take the loaded barbell off the rack and squat down until the barbell on your back taps the safety bars.

For the first set of partial squats, set the safety bar so that you will be doing about a one quarter squat. This will enable you to use some weights that are very heavy for you. See the picture below for the approximate depth of a ¼ squat.

The exercise is performed as follows: take the bar off the rack as if you were going to do a regular squat. Walk back to the starting position. Remember, do this with minimum number of steps. When you are set up and ready to squat, begin your descent as if you were going to do a full squat.

You will only descend until the weight taps the safety bars. At that point, stand erect and do one more repetition.

Keep the weight under control at all times. Just because you have a safety cage around you is no reason to get sloppy.

You will do **4 sets of 2 reps** with the safety bars set at the ¼ squat position. You will begin with a weight that is slightly above your 1 rep max full squat, and increase the weight by 3-5% of your 1 rep max on each set.

DO NOT do more than 2 reps in each set. You are training your body to put out maximum force and control a very heavy weight.

When you have placed the bar back on the rack, you should lower the safety bars by one hole. You will then do **2 sets of 2 reps** at this height.

When you lower the safety bars, you will not be able to use as much weight as you did on the first set. Find your starting weight by taking about 60% of your 1 rep maximum and seeing if you can descend and touch the safety bars with proper form. From there, you will find weights that you can do for 2 sets of 2 reps.

One of the strongest men of all time, the late Paul Anderson, used the cage to build his squatting to phenomenal levels. One of his special routines was to use the cage to work down progressively lower and lower with weights that he could only quarter squat at the beginning.

This is an extremely effective training technique, but requires a lot of effort over several months.

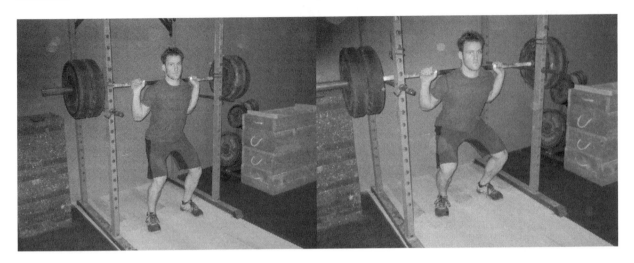

Beginning -Take the bar off the rack **Squat down and touch the safety bars**

The partial squat in the power rack will put a significant load on your central nervous system. If you have not done heavy training before, you will find that the few repetitions you perform in the cage will really tax you. It will take some time to build up your capacity to do a lot of work with really heavy weights.

Set the safety bars one hole lower, squat down, tap the safety bars, and return to erect position

The Deep Pause Squat

The second movement in this cycle trains is designed to promote explosiveness. This is the "Deep Pause" squat.

In this exercise, you will take a weight that is light for you (begin at 50% of your maximum) and descend to the lowest squat position you can. At that point, literally "pull" yourself deeper into the squat using your hip flexor muscles.

Keep your body tension, and remain in perfect squatting position. When you are in the deepest position you can reach, hold yourself there for a count of 5, then accelerate upward to a standing position *as fast as you can.*

You will be doing **4 sets of 2 reps**.

The two keys to success in this movement are: 1) pausing for a count of 5 in the deep position, and; 2) accelerating out of the bottom of the squat *as fast as you can*. Keep proper form throughout this movement.

There will be a strong temptation to accelerate out of the bottom by raising your hips first. You need to drive out of the bottom with your chest coming up first to get the benefit of this movement.

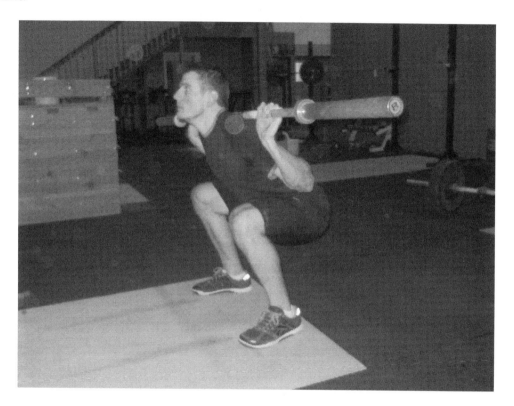

Deep Position – Ready for Rapid Ascent

Assistance Exercises:

Good Morning Exercise – This movement will really strengthen your posterior power chain...better known as the glutes, hamstrings and lower back. It can look like a squat gone terribly wrong, but in reality it is a great power builder.

You begin by taking a *light* weight off the squat rack with the bar in the same position you would use for a regular squat. Step back and set your feet wider than shoulder width. At that point, you bend forward at the waist until your torso is just above parallel position with the floor. Keep your back flat and flexed with a slight arch in your lower back. To keep your balance, bend your knees slightly. When you are bent forward the place where your torso is just above parallel, return to the starting position.

I emphasize *starting with a light weight*, since this movement can really surprise you if you have not done it before. It will put a huge stress on the hamstrings, and most people are not ready for doing hard work with their hamstrings through a full range of motion.

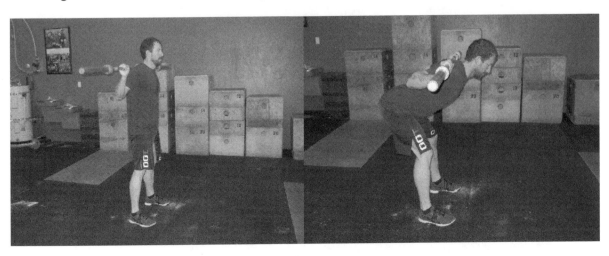

Good Morning – Starting Position   **Good Morning – Low Position**

You need to *insure* that you are doing the good morning exercise *through the full range of motion*. Be certain that you bend over at the waist, and lower your chest until your trunk is slightly above parallel to the floor. This means that you have *bent over almost 45 degrees* from the waist. I emphasize this because *so many people "cheat" on exercises by cutting the depth or range of motion*. If you want to get strong never "cheat" by cutting depth or doing the easy range of motion. Always do a movement through the full range of motion.

To insure that you do the good morning movement correctly, begin with a light weight. Even if you begin with a *really* light weight, if you consistently practice the movement correctly, you will be amazed at how strong you can become. This is one of those "big kid" exercises that build *real* strength and power. You need to do it correctly to get results.

To reinforce my point, the good morning exercise has become a standard movement for building back, hip and posterior leg strength in NFL weight training facilities. Competitive powerlifters have used it for decades with great results. But, you almost never see it done in "regular" gyms.

When you first do the good morning exercise, first work on mastering the movement, then begin adding weight. Start with **2-3 sets of 8-10 reps.** When you begin, you should select a weight that you can do easily for 10 reps. As you get more capable with the movement, you increase the weight, and keep the reps at 10. When you get stronger, and no longer have issues with balance or depth of the movement, go for heavier weights, more sets, and fewer reps.

Squat Cycle #3 – Elastic Band Training

One of the greatest assets to building a big squat are elastic training bands. In this program, I'll show you two of the best training band exercises that will add a huge amount to your power.

Elastic training bands come in a variety of sizes. In this program you will begin using bands that are intermediate in strength. When you have gained experience with using the bands, you can be more aggressive and use heavier bands.

In this program you will be doing regular squats, but with the elastic training bands working on the loaded bar as well. You will do all of these movements in a squat cage in order to string the bands properly, and for your own safety.

Upper Band Squat –

Begin by attaching the training bands to upper bracket of the squat cage at approximately the position where you will set up to do the squat. Attach the bands to the bar between the first barbell plate, and the inside collar. These are shown in the photographs below.

When you take the bar off the rack, the bands will be slack and provide no real change in the way the weight feels. However, as you descend, the bands will get tight and begin to take some of the weight off the bar. What this means is that you will be able to handle a much heavier weight in a deep squat position.

As the weeks go by and you practice this routine, you will be able to handle a very large weight at the top of the lift because it gets "lighter" as you descend. In the early going, it is best if you experiment and discover what weights you can manage. You will find that you can add weight rapidly to this exercise once you are used to how the weight "unloads" as you descend.

To do the exercise, begin with a weight that you can do 3 to 5 unassisted reps with. Attach the bands to the weigh and the squat cage as shown. Take the bar off the rack as if you were going to do a regular squat, take a deep breath and hold it, then descend as you would normally.

As you descend you will find that the weight becomes "lighter" as the bands stretch. How much lighter will depend on the strength of the bands you use and how much tension is placed on them. Each set of bands seems to be different, so assume that any estimate you make about the amount of weight lifted by the band will be approximate.

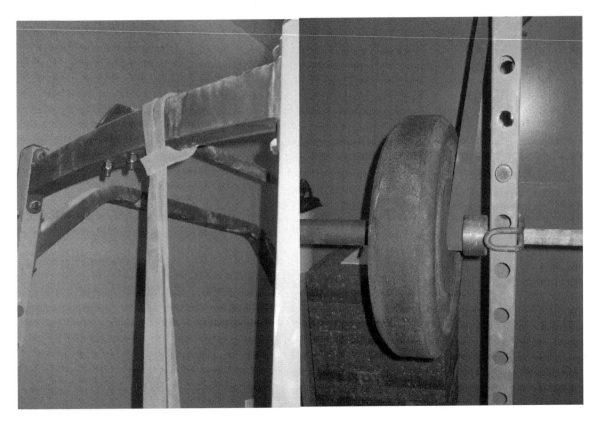

Proper way to attach band to the rack.

Proper way to attach band to the weight.

Do 3 sets of 3 reps and 1 set of 2 reps, increasing the weight on the bar each time.

The pictures below show how to do the lift with bands attached to the top of the squat cage.

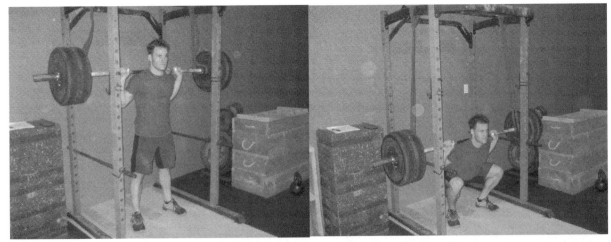

Starting Position: bands without tension

Bottom position: bands under max tension

Exercise #2 – Bands pull down

In this exercise, you will reverse the position of the bands, so that they pull the weight *down*. This exercise activates all of the muscles that work to keep you stable when doing the squat. This allows you to control more weight with the bar on your back.

The first thing you do is attach the elastic bands to either a safety bar at the bottom of the squat cage, or to a heavy dumbbell. See the pictures below to see examples of this.

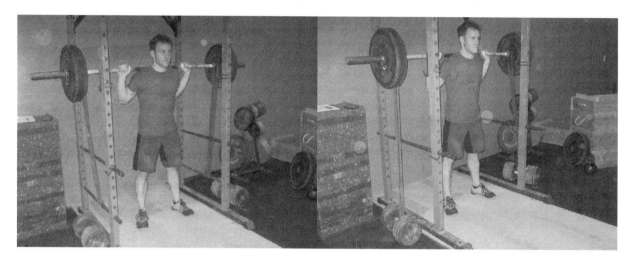

Bands attached to safety bars on the rack   **Bands attached to heavy dumbbells**

The main purpose of this exercise is to help you get better control of the weight on your back. When you take the weight off the rack it will suddenly feel like it wants to go in every different direction. The elastic band will be fighting you for control of the bar. For this reason, *begin with a very light weight.*

Don't be fooled by using a light weight. The elastic band will always fight you for control. This will build your stability and support muscle structure. That is very critical when you handle big weights. It will also build a lot of explosive power in the top third of the squat. You will notice this when you lock out a heavy weight.

As you get more skilled at controlling the weight, you can put more weight on the bar. However, the weight you use in this exercise should never go about 40-50% of your one rep maximum.

Do 6 sets of 2 reps. - This will tax your support muscles in ways you may not be used to. When you get fatigued, accidents can happen. Never be sloppy or casual about performing this movement.

Dumbbell Band Squat –

This exercise is designed to really activate your support muscle system through the entire range of the squat. Quite simply, this exercise is a regular squat with dumbbells or kettlebells hanging from elastic bands on the end of the squat bar.

Load the squat bar with a light weight as the weights hanging from the bands will bounce throughout the exercise and have you constantly working to stabilize the bar.

Do 2 sets of 3 reps with this exercise.

The pictures below show how to hang the weights from the end of the bar, and how the exercise is performed.

The weight should not touch the floor during this exercise. The bands can be doubled over to shorten them if touching the floor at the bottom is a problem.

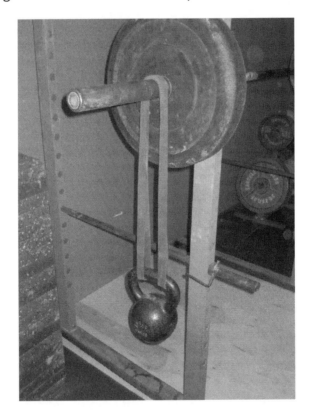

Hanging weight from the end of the bar

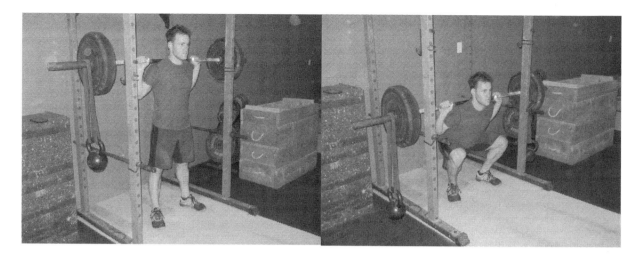

Starting Position   **Deep position: weight should not touch floor**

This exercise will pay off in terms of developing a lot of stability and explosiveness from all positions in the squat. Because you use light weights, you can do a few sets of this movement any time you feel the need to work on your stability during the lift.

Assistance Exercises

Kettlebell Goblet Squat – This exercise is great for building powerful stabilizer muscles, a strong core and great balance. In short, this movement gives a lot of payback for the effort. You also get a great stretch in the hips, glutes and lower back.

Begin standing upright and take a moderately heavy kettlebell in two hands, gripping it "by the horns" (opposite sides of the handle) as shown in the picture below. Keeping your chest up, your back flat with a slight arch in the lower back, descend into a deep squat as shown in the photo. When you have hit rock bottom, return to the standing position.

You should do **3 sets of 8-10 repetitions** with the goblet squat. When you can do 10 reps, increase the weight and go back to doing 8 reps.

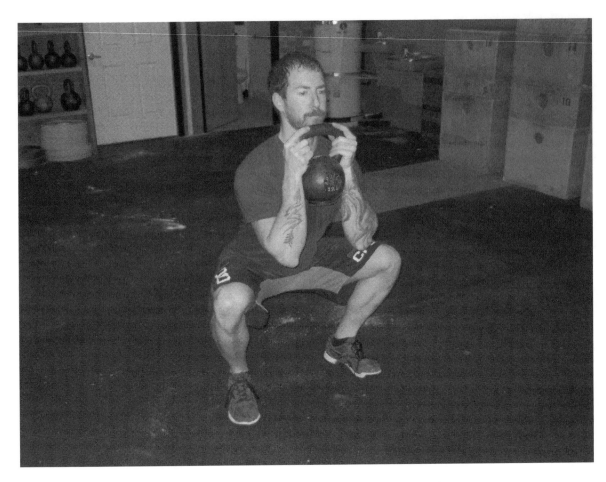

Kettlebell Goblet Squat – Bottom position

Hanging Leg Raise – Toes to Bar style – As noted earlier, a strong core is critical to building a powerful body, and a big time squat. This version of the hanging leg raise is more demanding than the ones used earlier in this course, and will give you super strength as well as a boost in your athleticism.

You should grasp a chin up bar that is high enough so that your feet do not touch the ground. Hang from a chin up bar as shown, and rapidly raise your fully extended legs until you are able to touch the chin up bar with your toes. You will tilt your pelvis toward the direction of the leg raise, and tighten you abs to bring your legs up. You should touch the chinning bar with your toes, and then drop your legs back to the starting position.

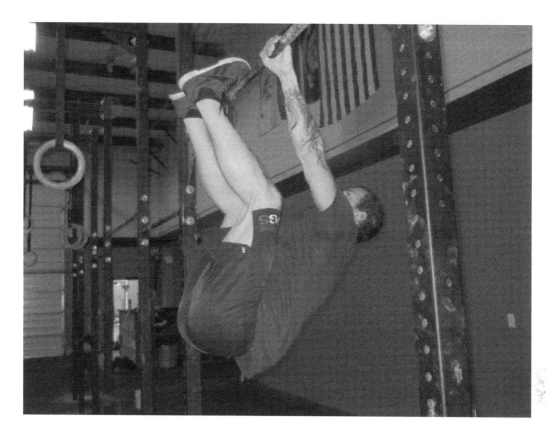

Hanging Leg Raise – Toes touching the bar

You will find that you fully engage your gore, your arms and shoulders doing this movement. It is difficult, and you may not initially be able to touch the bar with your toes more than a few times during the set of exercises. Keep pulling your toes as high as you can. Over time you will get stronger, and this movement will become routine for you.

Begin by doing **3 sets of 5 to 8 reps.** You should work up to doing 8 rep sets as soon as you can. When you are able to do 3 sets of 8 reps, switch to **2 sets of 12-15 reps.**

Squat Cycle #4 - Box Squats and Front Squats

Now that you have finished a second peaking cycle, and have a new 1 rep max squat in the books, you should give your body a break and work with lighter weights for a while. You will also notice that doing heavy squats has increased your other lifts, as your overall body strength is going up.

In this phase of your training you will build power in those parts of the squat that are typically most difficult for all lifters; the bottom of the squat, and the "sticking point".

By giving your body some variation from regular squats, you will be able to keep fresh and enthusiastic while building your overall strength. Box squats are one of the best movements for building power while giving you a nice change.

Box Squats –

Box squats are an exercise where you put the bar on your back like a regular squat and actually sit down on a very sturdy box. The box will have to support not only your weight, but also the weight of the loaded bar. For this reason, you *must always* sit on something that is really strong. Regular chairs will probably be crushed and may get you injured.

Most gyms will have an assortment of things you can use to sit on. In the photographs the lifter is sitting on heavy duty blocks. You can also sit on metal stands used for jumping, barbell plates, or heavy duty boxes built for gym use.

Do this exercise in a power cage as shown in the photographs. If you don't have a cage, be certain to use spotters because you may not be able to get up with a heavy weight.

Position the boxes as shown in the photograph. You will be taking the weight off the rack and backing into squatting position. When you first try this movement, experiment with a very light weight so that you get the feel for where you place the boxes so that you don't trip over them.

Set the safety bars about 6 inches below where the bar will be at its lowest point in your box squat. If you can't get up with a weight, you can simply bend forward at the waist and set it on the safety bars.

When the boxes and safety bars are properly positioned, you are ready to begin doing the exercise.

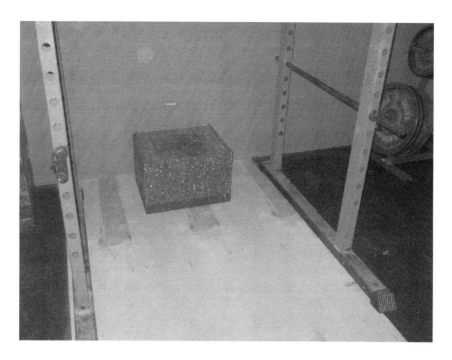

Box positioned in power rack

Box squats are done at different heights. You will have to adjust the height of the boxes as you do different sets of box squats. The blocks shown in the photograph can be stacked on top of one another to change heights. If you don't have stacking blocks, you will have to switch out boxes to get different heights. It will depend on what you have available in your training facility.

Group 1 – Box set <u>below</u> parallel – Group 2- Box <u>above</u> parallel - Your first sets of box squats will be done *below parallel.* Select a box or platform that will allow you to sit down with the bar on your back and is at least 2 inches below parallel. When the box is in position, take a practice rep without any weight on the bar to be certain that the boxes are set in the right place, and you don't have any problem sitting down on them. Now you are ready to begin.

Take a deep breath and hold it until you have squatted and come back to the starting position.

This is the technique for doing the box squat. Take the weight off the rack, and descend until your glutes contact the box. *At that point you will <u>sit down</u> as if you were in a chair.* You will relax your legs (somewhat) and sit upright. You then lean forward slightly and go back up to the starting position.

Look at the pictures carefully and see how the lifter has positioned his body in each part of the exercise.

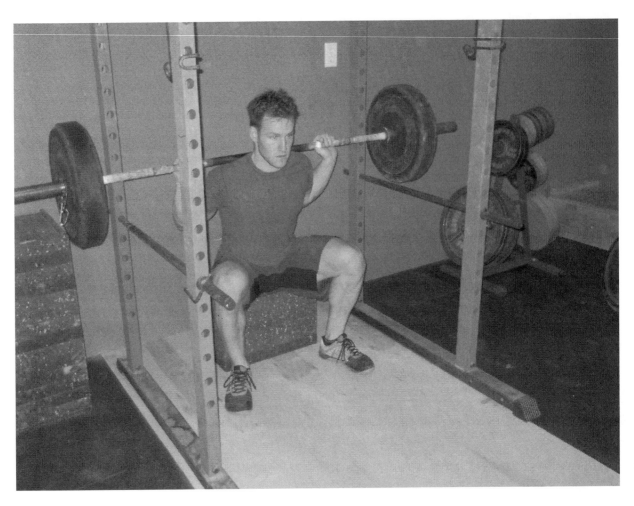

Sitting on the box below parallel

You can see that the lifter keeps his chest up, back flat and abs tight while sitting on the box. Do *not* allow your back to round or "roll over" at any point in this lift. This can be seen very clearly in the side view below.

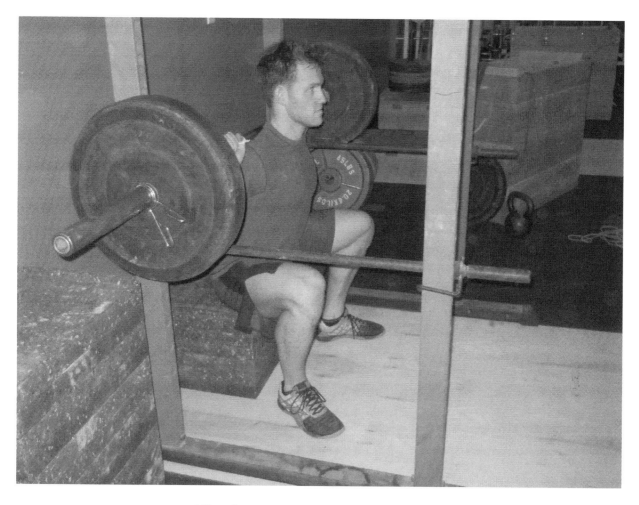

Lifter in proper position below parallel

The photo above shows the lifter sitting back on the box. To come back to the standing position, bend forward at the waist *slightly*, and come up with your chest coming up first. There will be a temptation to start coming up by throwing your rear end upward. Don't do that! Keep the same strict form you would use coming out of the bottom of a regular squat and this exercise will really help you build big power.

Box Squat

You will be doing box squats at two different heights: one below parallel, and one just above parallel. You will do **5 sets** of box squats at each height. Here is how you will select the weights to use:

> **Box below parallel:**
>
> > Set 1 – Light weight – 5 reps
> >
> > Set 2 thru 5 – Increase the weight to 70% of max – 2 reps

Box above parallel:

    Set 1 – Relatively easy set – 5 reps

    Set 2 – Increase to about 70% effort – 3 reps

    Set 3 – increase to about 80% effort – 1 rep

    Set 4 – Decrease to about 70% effort – 3 reps

Selecting weights that will work for you will require experimenting. Because the exercise may be new to many of you, it is important that you not start training with weights too heavy for you. This leads to quickly halting progress. You should experiment with weights to see what works best for you.

Always remember – your goal is to make progress over time, not exhaust yourself in one workout. Putting out all you have should only be done at those times when you are focusing on setting personal bests.

The Front Squat

The second exercise in this cycle is the front squat. This is one of the movements that Olympic weight lifters and Cross Fit enthusiasts train all the time, and is virtually ignored by everyone else. It is a great exercise for building a really powerful core. As such, it is one of the best ab exercises ever devised.

If you have not done this movement before, you should study the pictures to see how the bar is supported across the front of the shoulders. You should be resting the bar on what feels like a "shelf" across the collar bones and frontal deltoids. *You should not be supporting the bar with your hands or wrists.*

Gripping and supporting the bar across the shoulders is one of the things that seems to cause people the most problem in learning to do the front squat. The best way to get used to practicing this movement is to begin working with an empty bar and gradually add weight until you have mastered the proper technique.

When you take the bar across the front of your shoulders, you should begin with a grip that is slightly wider than your shoulders. Move forward under the bar, raise your elbows, *and extend your shoulders forward.* By moving your shoulders forward, you create the "shelf" on which the bar will rest.

Keep your elbows up, roughly parallel to the floor. Many of you will have to allow the bar to rest across the front of your shoulders, with only your fingertips in contact with the bar. See the picture to see how this looks.

Some of you will be able to keep a regular grip on the bar. This requires a lot of flexibility in the hands and wrists. (I do it this way because I learned how to do it at age 14 and have been doing it this way for the last 60 years). Either grip works.

Learning proper front squat technique will enable you to develop some serious upper body strength. You will also get a really nice look around the waist, as this lift builds a trim and very powerful mid-section.

You begin this lift by taking the bar off the rack and standing upright as shown in the picture below.

You can see that the bar is resting across the lifter's upper chest area, the elbows are elevated and parallel to the floor, the back is flat, and the feet are set slightly wider than shoulder width apart. The lifter is now ready to descend.

Take a deep breath and hold it until you have come all the way back to the starting position.

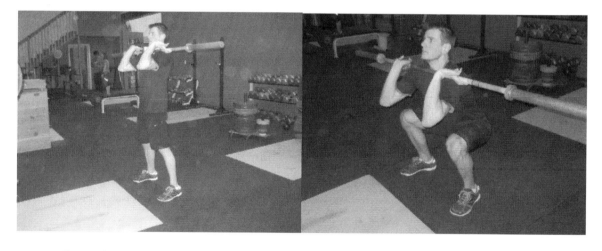

Front Squat - Starting position   **Front Squat –Deep position**

The first move is to push the buttocks back as if you were going to sit down. We have already discussed why you don't want to bend your knees forward. Descend into a low squat position, and *keep your head <u>slightly</u> up.* You should select a spot on the wall across from you, and focus your eyes on it.

Keeping your head slightly up and your upper arms parallel to the floor will keep your back straight, and prevent rounding the back.

When you have reached the lowest point in your front squat (well below parallel), you should power up out of the bottom and return to the standing position. You can release the breath when you are almost back to the starting position.

You will do **4 sets.** As in the box squat, you will have to experiment to see what weights you can effectively use as you learn this lift.

    Set 1 – Lightest weight – **5 reps**

    Set 2 – Select a weight that you could do 5 reps with – **3 reps**

    Set 3 – Same weight – **3 reps**

    Set 4 – Weight used on set 1 – **3 reps**

The purpose of doing an initial front squat routine is twofold; first learning how to do it properly, and secondly getting the full benefit of this demanding movement. If this is a new lift for you, or you have not practiced it extensively, take the time to learn how to do it well. This is one training movement that will pay huge dividends in both strength and appearance.

If you have been doing front squats before, you can work on perfecting your technique, and be more aggressive when it comes to the weights you use.

Assistance Exercises

Kettlebell swings –Alternating Hands –

A variation of the kettlebell swing that creates solid conditioning and good coordination is one where you alternate grip hands on each rep. As in the regular kettlebell swing, you swing the bell back between your legs as if you were hiking a football. You then suddenly drive the bell upwards using your hips, glutes and hamstrings. Your arms should not provide any force in driving the bell upward.

In the alternating hand variation, you will drive the bell upward to the point where it becomes stationary, then let go of it with one hand and grab the handle with the other. Then allow the bell to swing back between your legs while gripping with the other hand. You alternate the hand you use to grip the bell on each swing.

This produces a powerful "side-to-side" stress on your core. You will find that the alternating hand form of the swing requires a lot of coordination and focus.

You should not allow the bell to drift too far out in front of you, as that will make the hand exchange more and more difficult as you swing the bell. Keep the arc of the bell relatively close to your body so that you don't have to "reach" for the bell each time you change hands. The ideal arc would be one where the "catching" arm is slightly bent.

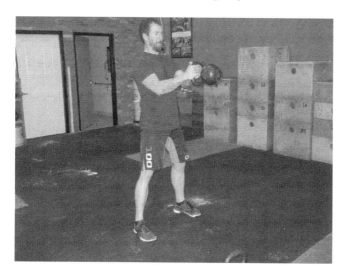

Alternate hand Kettlebell swing – top position

Remember that you should get the power from this movement from snapping your hips forward, and driving the bell up with this power. You should feel the effort coming from your abs, glutes and hamstrings. If you feel it coming from your lower back, you are doing the movement wrong.

Squat Cycle #5 – Peaking Cycle

Powerlifting competitors use a wide variety of "peaking" programs to increase their maximum lifts. This is a "peaking" program that you can do for **8 weeks.** The basic idea is that you will concentrate your effort into sets where you begin the cycle doing 3 reps, then go to 2 and ultimately to 1 rep.

You will also do two assistance exercises that will help build explosiveness into your squatting.

Exercise #1 – Full Squat – Peaking Cycle

The first six weeks of the cycle, you will be doing 4 sets of squats each training session. The big difference from previous routines is that you will *alternate one heavy and one light workout each week.* That way you will essentially do **one heavy training session each week.** The second session will be to help you build explosiveness and muscular endurance.

The squat routine looks like this:

Week 1-3

Heavy Day – Squat

    Set 1: 70% of 1RM – 3 reps

    Set 2: 80% of 1RM - 3 reps

    Set 3: 85% of 1RM – 3 reps

    Set 4: 80% of 1RM – 3 reps

Assistance lifts:

    Dumbbell or Kettlebell Lunge – 2 sets of 10 reps

    Dimmil (partial) Deadlift – 2 sets of 15 reps

Week 4-6

Heavy Day – Squat

    Set 1: 75% of 1RM – 2 reps

    Set 2: 85% of 1RM – 2 reps

Set 3: 95% of 1RM - 1 rep

Set 4: 85% of 1RM - 1 rep

Assistance work: Same as week 1-3

Week 7

Heavy Day:

Set 2: 95% of 1RM – 1 rep

Set 3: 102% of 1RM – 1 rep

NO assistance work in week 7 of the peaking cycle

Week 8

Contest or personal best attempt.

After warming up do single reps with:

85% of 1RM

103% of 1RM

107% of 1RM -or your best estimate of what you can do

You should do all full squats with perfect technique. This will insure that you get the maximum training effect from the program. Once your technique begins to erode, you limit the chances you have for doing really heavy squats.

Assistance Exercises:

The Dumbbell of Kettlebell Lunge

The lunge is one of the great exercises for building strength and power in the legs, hips core and back. It is also an exercise that is almost always done with horrible technique, and is thus of little or no value. You, of course, will do it correctly and get monster strong.

If you have been frequenting "regular gyms" you probably see people doing lunges like shown in the picture immediately below. These are worse than useless, and are likely to get you hurt. Doing lunges like this will insure that you never get any real benefit from the exercise.

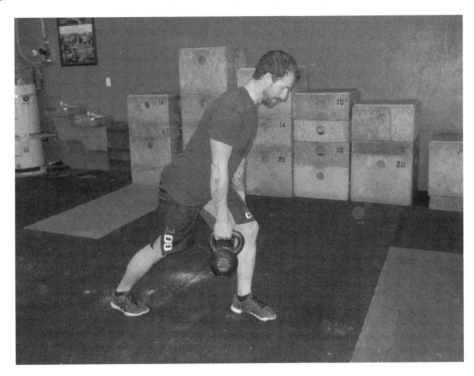

A "Results Free" version of the Lunge

Before showing you how to do the lunge correctly, I want to point out some of the major problems with the "results free" version shown above.

First of all, there is no depth to the lunge, so there is no training benefit to the hips, core or upper leg. The model is bent forward, so there is extra stress on the lower back and neck. Finally, the shoulders are rounded so that the neck and upper back are in poor alignment. The foot spacing is so narrow that there is no challenge that requires developing better balance or coordination. If a person takes tiny steps and does not go deep into the lunge, they can boast about lifting much bigger weights than they could do if they did the exercise correctly. This is of course a complete illusion.

There are more problems with this example, but by now you can see that this type of lunge NOT what *you* want to be doing. Doing the lunge correctly will yield a ton of benefits in strength and athleticism.

Let's start by insuring that your trunk is upright. You never want to bend forward <u>at any time</u> when doing lunges. The second issue is the length of the stride; thus how deep you go in the bottom portion of the lunge. Look at the photos below and see how a proper lunge is performed.

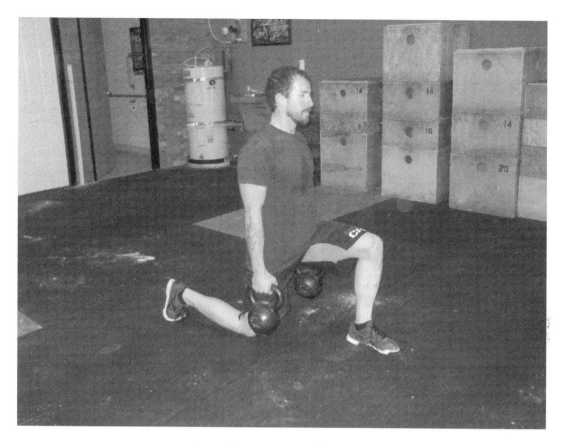

Proper form for kettlebell/dumbbell lunge

You should begin in a standing position with a kettlebell or dumbbell in each hand. Take a step forward with your right leg so that you descend into a position where the top of your right thigh is parallel to the floor. Your trunk should be absolutely vertical, and the weights should hang down at your sides directly alongside your hips.

When you step forward, you immediately confront the issue of maintaining balance when you go into the deep position (also called the "split"). If you lead with your right leg, then your step forward should be a *slightly* to the right rather than straight ahead. This will allow you to keep your balance while holding weights in the split position. You should experiment with the foot position that works best for you by doing the lunge without weights.

You should come out of the split by straightening your front (right) leg. You then bring the front (right) leg *back* to the rear (left) leg. When you do this, you will be standing on exactly the same spot you were when you began the exercise.

Some versions of the lunge have you bringing the back leg up to the front leg. This means that you "walk" around the exercise area. You can do this if you want, but the stationary version of the lift creates fewer requirements for training space. There is no particular benefit for doing the "walking" version of the lunge.

Do lunges **2 sets of 10 reps. Each step is a rep.** That means that you will be doing 5 reps with each leg on each set.

Begin with a weight that is relatively easy to manage. It is *far more* important that you master the proper technique for lunging than it is that you create an illusion that you can handle artificially high weights. Increase the weights when you can do so and keep perfect form.

The Dimmil (Partial) Deadlift

The assistance exercises in this program are probably new to you. Each of them builds a major component of your overall body power. The first is named for a legendary master of the squat, the late Matt Dimmil. He invented this exercise back at the Westside Barbell Club in Columbus, Ohio back in the 1980's. This is a "partial deadlift", but done in a very specific way in order to really build up the posterior power chain: your glutes, hamstrings, hips and lower back.

Like all other power exercises, the technique on this movement is very important. You begin by loading a *very light* weight on the barbell. For example, the Columbus studs who squatted over 900 lbs would load the bar to 225. If you are a 400-pound squatter, you should load the bar to about 135. There is NO real advantage to be gained by using unusually heavy weight in this exercise. The purpose is to build *speed and explosiveness.*

As the weight is light, you will use a grip where both palms are turned inward toward the body. Set your feet at the spacing you use for a squat. Grab the bar so your arms hang straight down....no wide grips, no narrow grips. Stand up with the bar hanging at arm's length. You are ready to begin the exercise.

You lower the bar to the midpoint of your shins. <u>Do not</u> lower the bar all the way to the floor. When you reach the midpoint of the shins, stand erect *very rapidly.* You should impel the bar upward by driving your hips forward and straightening your legs at the same time. Your arms *do not* contribute anything to moving the bar. They are merely "ropes" you use to hang on to the bar.

When you reach the top, immediately drop the bar quickly back to the midpoint of the shin, and then explosively stand erect. You will repeat this 20 times!

The key to success in this exercise is to be *fast and explosive*. There is little benefit to doing this exercise slowly.

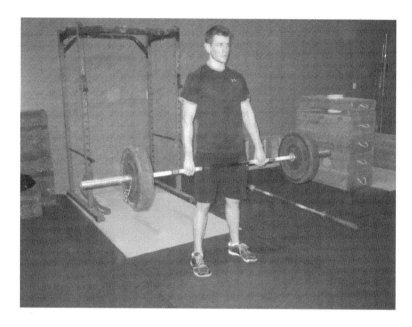

Starting position

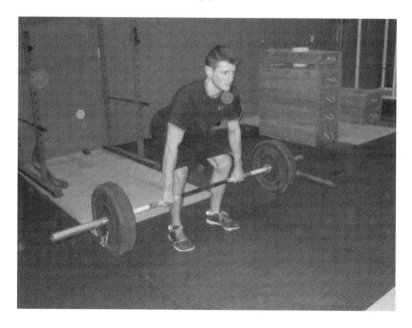

Low Position at mid-shin- <u>*don't*</u> touch the floor

Recovery Prior to Attempting Your Personal Best

In the last two weeks of this cycle, you will stop doing all assistance exercise. You are saving up for the maximum effort you will put out in Week 8...a personal best for one rep.

You should always be aware of the propensity for lots of lifters to over train and burn up needed energy in the gym, rather than getting a superior single lift. If you are a real "gym rat", you will probably know lots of lifters who failed to reach a goal because they didn't pay attention to recovering and doing what is *really* needed to lift big weights.

Perhaps the most common reason to miss making a personal best attempt is that the lifter has done *way too much work in the last weeks before attempting a maximum lift.*

The biggest single thing that will help you get a new personal best, or max lift is <u>getting the proper rest and recovery in the week or ten days before attempting the record lift.</u>

Let me tell you what some of the greatest strength coaches of all time have said about this.

I'll paraphrase the great Louie Simons who said "There is *nothing* you can do to get stronger in the week before a (max lift attempt), but there certainly is a <u>lot you can do to get weaker</u>".

The great Dan John said "Lifting heavy weights will not make your strong. Lifting heavy weights <u>and recovering</u> will make you very strong."

Rest and recovery is absolutely essential if you are going to become the best you can possibly be.

Chapter 7

Bench Press: THE Most Popular Lift

It will come as no surprise that the bench press is the most popular exercise in the world. If you go to any gym, you will see almost everyone in the place will include the bench press at some point in their workout.

The bench press is a great way to build upper body strength. It is also the second of three lifts in a powerlifting meet.

I suspect that the lift is popular because it gives a great workout for the arms, chest and shoulders and *appears* relatively easy to do.

Being an astute reader, you will note that I put the word "appears" in italics above. This is because doing something that looks like a bench press is a movement that can be done by anyone. Doing a bench press that mobilizes all your strength and power is an entirely different matter.

In the section on squatting, I went into a lot of detail about how to get the most power into the movement. That is precisely what I'll do for the bench press.

Begin by assuming that almost every bench press you ever see done in the typical gym is performed with terrible form and never comes close to the lifters maximum potential. If you have been lifting for some time, you may have to start bench pressing from scratch to eliminate your bad habits.

Don't expect the personal trainers to know anything about competition style bench pressing unless they compete regularly. In my experience fewer than 1 in 100 trainers have any idea of how to coach a competition bench press.

But…. don't despair. Pay really close attention to all the things I tell you, and practice them until you have mastered them. Working *smart* on the bench press and developing excellent technique will allow you to lift some really serious iron, reach your full potential, and all according to the very strict rules that define a legal competition lift.

Remember, having bad technique will mean that you automatically limit how far you can progress. Good technique is both to provide maximum mechanical advantage, and to insure that there are uniform standards for doing a competition lift.

In the next dozen pages, I'll take you through every detail you *need to master* in order to become the best bench presser you can be. Most of you will not have seen a dozen pages devoted to performing a lift that seems so simple. However, by now you know that lifting serious iron is not simple….so let's get to the step by step process of performing the bench press.

Proper Technique: Step by Step

Getting tight

The first thing you need to rivet into your mind is that <u>*the bench press is a whole body lift.*</u> This is not simply a lift to "develop the chest and shoulders".

Your objective is to *recruit* every ounce of power you can from you whole body. Remember, isolation is just the opposite of what you want to do.

To be effective in the bench press, you have to have your entire body tight as it is possible to make it. Any relaxed muscles will cause you to lift much less than your potential.

If you don't get your entire body tight…..almost nothing else I tell you will matter.

Like the squat, you will go through the process of getting your entire body tight *before* you take the bar off the support rack.

Setting up

A proper set up begins *before* you sit down on the bench. There are some variations in the way top notch lifters get on the bench. I'll describe one that is easy to do, and can be completely effective for as long as you lift heavy.

Assume the bar is loaded to the weight you are going to lift. Assuming that you are lifting without a supportive shirt (bench shirt) tighten your lifting belt before you lie down on the bench. I'll discuss support equipment in a section below. For now, assume that you tighten your belt before you get on the bench.

Stand over the end of the bench with your back to the bar, and position your feet so that when your body is on the bench, your feet will be on the floor back of your knees. Look at the picture below to see the foot position you want. The toes will line up with the front of your knees.

While standing, tighten your abs, back, and shoulders. Sit down on the bench and slide your body away from the bar until your knees are even with or slightly ahead of your toes. Tighten your glutes, legs and feet at this point. Dig the balls of your feet into the floor. Try to pinch your glutes together as hard as you can while flexing your abs. Your back should be arched with your butt on the bench.

If you have shorter legs, you can use barbell plates under each foot to enable you to set your feet properly. In lifting contests, you can request blocks to be set at the end of the bench so that you can position your feet properly.

In the picture, the lifter has his feet flat on the floor. Some lifting associations allow you to be up on your toes. If you are going to compete, it is important that you know what rules apply to your association.

I have always preferred the flat footed position, since I felt it gave me the most solid base of support. This position is considered competition legal in all of the lifting associations.

When you lie back on the bench, insure that your butt is completely tight and in contact with the bench.

Take a deep breath and hold it.

Very important: once you are on the bench, move your feet back toward your head. This has the effect of tightening your back and the rear side of your legs. You should feel this a lot in your lower back. The effect should be like a big spring that is tight. When you lower the bar to your chest, this tight "spring" is a big part of the resistance that will help you drive the bar upward.

Most lifters use an arch in their back, keeping their butt on the bench as this really helps staying tight. The amount of arch will vary person to person, but virtually everyone uses some arch.

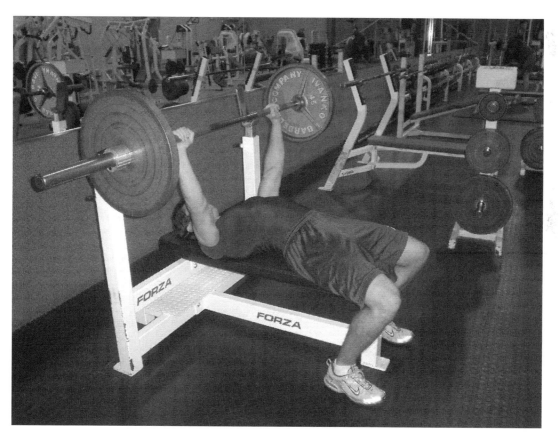

Perfect position for starting the Bench Press

Drive your shoulders into the bench, and push your shoulders down toward your toes. At this point your body should be *totally rigid*. *If a forklift picked you up, your position would not change in the slightest.*

Now, reach up and grasp the bar with the grip you intend to use in the lift. See the next section about grip spacing and technique. The bar should be on the rack slightly behind the top of your head.

As you grasp the bar, you tighten your arms. Begin by flexing your biceps (yes), and trying to crush the bar with your grip. Try to pull your upper arm into the shoulder socket and try to pull your forearm into your elbow socket.

Now that your entire body is completely tight, and you have a death grip on the bar, with your hands try to bend the lifting bar.

At this point you should be under maximum tension, and you are ready to take the bar from the rack.

The Grip

Grip technique is very important. Every major powerlifting association has rules about what grips are legal for competition. It is *critical* that you know these so that you train using legal grips.

The first thing you need to do is insure that your bar is marked at the proper places for you to place your grip. The most critical mark is 9.6 inches (29 cm) from each collar. Whatever grip you select, some part of your hand must cover this mark, or be inside of it. You cannot have a grip where the mark is exposed.

If you train with regulation powerlifting bars, there should be no problem. Most gyms will have bars that are marked somewhat randomly. Why this is the case, I have no idea, other than that the people who design exercise equipment must have no idea about the rules of powerlifting. Thus, markings are put on the bar for decoration.

You need to know precisely what the marks on your training bar actually mean. I advise taking a tape measure to the gym at least once and measuring the distance from the collar to the marking so you know where you can legally grasp the bar.

Finding out you have been training using an illegal grip width can cause you a lot of grief.

Now, when it comes to selecting the grip width you will use, the best one for you will depend on your unique leverages. This includes how long your arms are, how tall you are, and the shape of your torso.

Tall people will naturally take wider grips than short people. If you have not already found a preferred grip spacing, I would suggest that you experiment with different hand placement by adjusting it roughly ½ (1.5 cm) inch in a given direction, and train with it for a month. You should notice a difference (better or worse) in that time.

If you are just starting out, I would start using a grip that where the marking on the bar is in the middle of your hand. You can adjust in or out depending on how much power you are able to generate with different spacing.

Of course, if you are shorter than 5 ' 6" (167 cm) you should opt for a narrower grip to start. If you are taller than 6'2" (188 cm) you should opt for a wider starting point.

Grip width is not the only thing you need to address. How you wrap your fingers around the bar is both a rules issue and one where the alignment of the grip can maximize your ability to push.

International powerlifting federations require that all the fingers be wrapped around the bar, and that the "thumbs around" grip must be used. The "thumb less" grip (aka. The "suicide grip") cannot be used in competition.   This refers to holding the bar so that the thumb and the other fingers are all on the same side of the bar.

Another grip that cannot be used in competition is the "reverse" grip where you turn your palms so that instead of facing toward your feet, they face in the opposite direction.

This grip is quite risky, and I would advise that you avoid it completely. There is ample chance for the bar to slip out of either hand, and hit you in the face.

The way the bar sits in your hand is important.   You want the bar to rest in your hand so that when you push upward the bar is aligned directly over your forearm. The full force of your push upward will be slightly dissipated if you hand is bent backward at the wrist and the bar is positioned over empty space. This happens when you lay the bar across the center of your palm.

When you grip the bar, insure that the *heel of your palm opposite the thumb* is where you will push upward on the bar. The bar should lie in a slight diagonal so that it is over the heel of your palm, not directly across the center of your palm. Pressure on the heel of your palm causes your triceps to become fully engaged in the upward press.

This little trick comes from the Russians who perfected it in Olympic style lifting several decades ago. The crafty Russians found that moving the press upward with the bar on the heel of your hand made the triceps fire with maximal force. This provided an advantage to those lifters who used it.

In the era before powerlifting (1950's and 1960's) the "macho" lift was the standing military press. Bench pressing was mainly for bodybuilders. The man who could do a strict standing press with his body weight was considered a "stud".

Having done Olympic style lifting in that era, I can attest that doing a strict press with body weight was really hard. You can use this little grip trick in the bench press and get a boost to your press. It takes practice, but you will find that this grip can give you a few extra pounds on each lift.

The Lift Off and the Critical Role of Spotters

I always advise using a spotter to give you a lift off and help you if you miss a lift. Having the confidence that the spotter will help you out of any difficulty is worth many pounds when you are lifting heavy.

From a safety standpoint, a good spotter is worth their weight in gold. They can save your bacon if something goes wrong. If you work heavy, there is always a good chance that you will need to be bailed out.

If you are serious about wanting to develop a top flight bench press, having a good spotter during training is critical. The spotter is the person who will give you the lift off, do the referee calls, and insure that you don't get injured.

You can use a training partner as a spotter, or any person you regularly see at the gym who is willing to do the job. _You need to train them to do exactly what you want_, so that there is no chance of them getting crossed up, or not knowing what to do in a certain situation.

Depending on how heavy a weight you are lifting, you will use one or three spotters. For weights under 300 pounds, you can probably use only the middle spotter positioned right behind your head who will do the lift off for you. For weights over 300 pounds, (unless your spotter is a really big strong guy) I recommend using additional spotters on each end of the bar.

As a rule of thumb, I would suggest that as long as the middle spotter can easily deadlift the weight you are bench pressing, you can use one spotter. Once the weight gets above that, you need to go to three spotters.

The spotters on the end of the bar are there to catch and stabilize the bar if you lose control. They will literally "catch" a lift if you suddenly lose it. They then hold the weight in place until the middle spotter can grab the bar. Then the three spotters _and_ the lifter can lift the bar back to the rack.

In no case should a spotter on the end of the bar suddenly lift up on the bar. That could cause the weight to suddenly go wildly out of balance. The end spotters initial job is to catch the bar and stabilize it so that the "four of you" can lift it back on to the rack.

End spotters must hold their hands with interlocked fingers under the end of the bar as you lower it. It is mandatory that they use the interlocking finger grip, and follow the bars descent with their hands an inch or two below the end of the bar.

If they do not have their fingers interlocked positioned an inch or two under the bar while it descends, their presence is useless. When things go wrong on a heavy bench press, it happens so fast that no one on earth has quick enough hands to grab the bar before a serious injury could occur. I preach this because I have seen what happens when a lifter suddenly loses a heavy lift.

In one memorable case, the spotters were football players from an SEC school who spent a ton of time in the weight room. They were spotting for a guy lifting 400 in the bench press. The spotters on the end had their hands in front of them, but not interlocking fingers under the end of the bar. Suddenly the lifter lost control of the weight, and in the blink of an eye it had crashed down to a safety stand before the spotters could even react.

The safety stand was positioned just above the lifters neck. If the safety stand had not been there, the lifter might have been decapitated. At a minimum, he would have been seriously injured if not crippled.

Virtually no gym in the country has safety racks for bench press benches. The only reason they were in place in the event I just described was that it was part of a sanctioned competition that required the safety racks be in place.

The moral of this story is that you need to have competent spotters who know what they are doing if you plan to lift heavy.

Now for the all-important lift off.....

The middle spotter is the one who will do the lift off. The middle spotter should be in position before you get on the bench, and wait for you to get positioned to do the lift. When YOU are ready to take the bar, you need to signal the spotter to lift it off the rack for you.

The middle spotter should be standing behind your head at the middle of the bar when it sits on the rack. The spotter must have both hands on the bar in a position that does not interfere with the lifters grip.

This means, you need to be on the bench with your grip set and be prepared to take the bar.

You have to tell the middle spotter when you want him or her to hand you the bar.

Clearly telling the middle spotter when to lift the bar off the rack and hand it to you is really important. I have always found a "1-2-3" count works really well. On the count of 3, the spotter lifts the bar off the rack and helps you move it (almost instantly) to the stable lockout position above your face.

The spotter is not going to lift the whole weight. You need to be pressing upward on the bar so that the spotter only has to lift about half the weight loaded on the bar.

In a quick coordinated movement, the spotter lifts the bar up and together you position the bar at the stable lockout positon right above your face. At that point, you should have complete control of the weight held at arm's length. The spotter should quickly remove their hands from the bar at that point.

In a competition, the referee will not allow you to lower the bar to your chest until the spotter's hands are no longer in contact with the bar.

This is the starting point for the lift.

Lowering the Bar

To be ready to lower the bar, you should be motionless on the bench, and your entire body should be tight. You should drive your shoulders down toward your toes, and push your head into the bench. This keeps everything maximally tight.

Many lifting federations require that the referee tell you when to lower the weight. Normally this is the word "start". This is to insure that you have full control of the bar before beginning the lift.

Some federations allow you to lower the bar whenever you feel you are ready. In either case, you should practice the way you will perform the lift in a contest during your training. It is very difficult to suddenly start doing something in a contest that you have not practiced.

You should be holding a deep breath that you took before you got on the bench.

Lowering the bar correctly is a major part of building a big bench press. This is where you "load" all the muscles that will drive the bar upward.

The picture you should have in your mind is that the weighted bar is creating huge pressure in your personal hydraulic system. The lower the bar goes; the more pressure builds up in your body. When the bar is on the chest, your personal hydraulic system has been compressed to the maximum and is ready to explode the bar upward.

Lower the bar *slowly* under full control with every muscle in your body *tight.* The bar will come down in an arc, with the starting point being over your face, and the bottom point on the solar plexus or the bottom of the rib cage.

The pressure is building! You should be trying to bend the bar with your hands, and flex your biceps. This will add to the amount of power you can generate.

As you bring the bar down, your elbows should move into your sides until they are flush against your sides when the bar is on your chest.

Some people prefer to flare their elbows out during the bench press. This is more of a bodybuilding movement than a power movement as it has the pecs do the bulk of the work. It also puts extreme stress on the shoulder joint. Over time most lifters opt for the elbows into the sides as you can mobilize more muscle groups using this technique.

As the bar descends, pinch your shoulder blades together and load tension into your lats.

Keep pushing your shoulders down toward your toes, which is down and slightly toward the floor. Your abs should be pushing hard against your lifting belt. You should feel the pressure building throughout your body.

You should feel as if a giant hand is *forcing* the bar down to your chest. All your muscles are loading tension so that they will be ready to drive upward when the bar is on your chest.

You are holding your breath all the time the bar is lowering. The breath in your lungs will add to the compression and help you with the upward drive. Your entire body *must* be tense. If any part of it is relaxed, you will lose a huge amount of power…just like a leak in a balloon.

As I noted above, you are aiming to place the bar just at the bottom of your rib cage or slightly lower. Some lifting associations allow you to lower the bar to your stomach. This positions lower on the torso give you absolute maximum leverage for the push upward.

One of the biggest mistakes novices make is to lower the bar so that it touches the chest at the nipples. This position cuts out the powerful push you can get from the lats and all of the pecs. It also puts huge stresses on the shoulder joint Instead of recruiting power from the whole body, landing the bench press "high" on the chest means the lift is done only with the triceps and frontal deltoids.

Now you have the bar on your chest and are ready for the dreaded "pause". This separates the sheep from the lions pretty quickly.

The "Pause"

The biggest difference between the garbage style bench presses you see done in a typical gym, and a competition bench press is "the pause". In competition, you have to <u>hold the bench press bar motionless on your chest before pushing upward.</u> Competitive bench pressing is also more demanding because you must *wait* for the referee's signal to "press" before you can push the bar up.

The length of time you have to hold the bar will vary a bit from one lifting association to another. The interval is usually about 1 full second. This can seem like the better part of an hour if you are the one holding the bar.

Most recreational lifters use the "touch and go" style of bench pressing. That is the instant the bar touches the chest, the lifter reverses thrust and drives the bar to arm's length. This style of pressing is **_never_** allowed in competition.

There may be some exceptions to this in some remote and lame corner of the lifting kingdom. "Touch and Go" bench pressing may be allowed in contests sponsored by *The Bench Press Trophy Give Away Federation.* None of the major federations will allow touch and go lifting.

Therefore...it is imperative that you practice the pause, because without it, the referees will give you a "no lift" judgement.

It is best to remember that you will *always* do the things in a meet that you do in practice. You can't suddenly start using long pauses if you have not practiced them over and over so that they are automatic.

The first thing you need to practice is getting the bar motionless on your chest.

This means *nothing* is moving. There is no wobble in the bar, no motion from the hands, and no movement from one side to another. Your feet are also still. Your body and the bar must look like they are *frozen in a still photograph*.

You should practice "motionless" with a light bar so that you know what it feels like. This is what you need to duplicate with your competition lifts.

The next thing you need to do is practice the pause itself.

Begin with a light weight and keep the bar motionless on your chest for a count of 5. Gradually work up in weight until you can hold 60% of your 1 rep max for a count of 5. (You will note that the speed you count to 5 may get faster as the weights get heavier).

Having spent 22 years as a referee at the local and national level, and having seen thousands of bench presses in competition, I can assure you that many lifters get the bar to their chest and then spend some time trying to become "motionless". The good (and great) lifters bring the bar to the chest and are instantly motionless.

The quicker the bar is motionless, the quicker you will get the "press" command from the head referee.

Pressing off the Chest

Up to now you have been preparing for the big push upward. If you have done your work on the set up, lowering the bar, and the pause, the drive off the chest will be your reward.

When the bar is on your chest, your elbows are against your sides and the bar is completely stable and motionless. Your whole body is under maximum tension….a big spring ready to uncoil. You should never allow the bar to sink into your chest.

Keep your arms in at your sides in the bottom of the lift. This will activate the lats at the bottom and keep your triceps pushing full blast throughout the extension. As you press the bar further off your chest, you will begin to move your elbows out. This will feel like a natural groove for you.

This is a particularly relevant point for lifters over age 50 (and often much younger). Over the years of lifting, playing sports and just living, most of us accumulate some damage to the shoulder area.

In order to protect your shoulder as much as possible, I recommend that you use the bench pressing technique where you bring your arms in tight against your sides. You can still generate awesome power, but you don't put excessive stress on your shoulders by using the "elbows in" style of bench pressing.

After you have held the bar motionless on your chest, you get the command from the referee to "press".

Once you get the press command, *never* allow the bar to sink into your chest. This will get your lift disqualified (downward motion) …and it means you have relaxed somewhere.

Because you are holding the bar on your lower chest with your back arched, your initial push off the chest will be a bit toward your toes. In the initial moment of pushing the bar off your chest, you should feel the push in your lower back, lats, abs and glutes. Your abs should be pushing against your lifting belt. You should feel the upward push in the balls of your feet.

As it rises a few inches you will be pressing in a groove that gradually moves the bar move back toward your head. Remember, the bar goes down and up in an arc. You will feel the arc as it is the place where you have the greatest power.

Keep pushing your shoulders down toward your toes and into the bench. Your head should be driving back into the bench.

You will drive the bar upward following the same arc you did as you lowered it. This is the arc where you have the most power. It will move from your lower chest back toward your face as the bar moves upward.

Again, any relaxed muscle is like a leak in a balloon. There goes the power.

You have to keep your butt on the bench or the attempt will be a "no lift". However, you want to fully engage your feet, legs, abs and back on the push. Your abs should be pushing against your lifting belt. All should be lock down tight and all your energy should flow toward pushing the bar upward.

A few inches off your chest is where you find the dreaded "sticking point". This is where moving the bar shifts from one set of muscles to another. Keep driving your shoulders toward your toes, and recruit max power from your lats and back.

You should be trying to flex your biceps as the bar rises. To do this try to "pull" the lifting bar apart. Again, this movement recruits more and more muscles to the task of moving the bar.

Throughout the upward push, the bar should move evenly. At no time can the bar dip or go downward. If either hand goes down during the upward push, it is "no lift".

Your feet should never move once the upward press begins. Your whole body should be rigid.

When you near the completion of the lift, or the "lock out" phase, you should straighten your arms at the same time. An uneven lock out is reason for disqualification of the attempt in some lifting associations, but not in all.

When you are at the top of your lift, fully locked out, you can release your breath.

Wait for the referee to give the command "rack it", and then put the bar back on the rack. To cement this habit in your mind, during practice you should have the person spotting for you give the command.

When you get the "rack it" command, the middle spotter should grab the bar and assist you getting it back on the rack. If you have spotters on the ends of the bar, they should simply support the bar so that the four of you get it back to the rack with no problems.

At that point, you will have completed the lift.

Common Mistakes

The _most common mistake_ in bench pressing is _to have some part of the body relaxed when trying to drive the weight off the chest._

This typically begins with not getting tight before lifting the bar off the rack. It can also happen by relaxing some muscles during the lift.

The number one sign that something is relaxed is that the lifters _feet move_ at some point in the lift.

If the feet move at all, some muscle group is relaxed that should be tight. Even a little movement means that the body is not locked down tight. The feet should be driving into the floor the whole time the bar is going up or coming down. There is no way that any foot movement can happen if your feet are driving into the floor.

Any time you see any movement in the feet, you know the legs are relaxed, and the back is probably relaxed. Moving feet = power failure.

Another common mistake is not crushing the bar with your grip, or trying the bend the bar while you lift. In short, <u>not recruiting every muscle you can during the lift!</u>

Failing to do this means that the lifter is not recruiting all the muscle power they can from the arms, shoulders and upper back.

Failing to recruit strength stems from being taught to do a bench press by "going through the motion" of doing a bench press when first learning how to lift. The lifter learns how to use a *few* muscles to move the bar up and down. If the lift "looks like a bench press", the assumption is that it must *be* a bench press. No way!

By now you are aware that a heavy lift is not the same as a light lift even though they may look the same motion to a naïve observer.

Learning how to recruit power from every muscle in your body is *difficult*. It takes a lot of work to learn this and consistent practice to do regularly. Most people *"don't do difficult"*.

A third common mistake will sound a little weird, but in my observation is very common. This mistake is that as the weight gets heavier, some lifters technique falls apart. A lifter may be able to do perfect reps with 80% of their max, but as the weight gets heavier, they start getting spooked and revert to something of a panic response.

In my view this happens because the *mental stress* of moving very heavy lifts is very different than the stress associated with lifting light weights. Fear creeps in as the weight gets bigger.

This is a normal reaction and one related to self-preservation. After all, lowering a weight that is at (or above) your limit *should* cause you to be concerned. If you were not wary of big iron, you would be a dunce.

Using competent spotters goes a long way to relieving the worry about handling big weights during training or competition. You know as you set up to lift your max that your personal safety is not in jeopardy. That is why I stress the importance of having well trained and capable spotters for serious lifts.

There are some other common mistakes that can be lumped under the heading of "being sloppy" (as in half-assed) about the lift. These include:

- Placing the feet directly below the knees or out in front of the bench
- Starting to lower the weight to the chest without holding it steady at arm's length
- Allowing the bar to sink into chest on the bottom of the lift

- Butt comes off the bench at any point in the lift
- Moving any part of the body during the lift, other than the arms
- "Throwing" the weight back on the rack after completing a set
- Not using the same precise form, regardless of the weight on the bar
- Getting on the bench relaxed and then trying to get tight
- Not fully locking out each bench press
- Relaxing during some part of the set
- Training "to failure" on one or more sets

By now you have figured out that there are <u>lots of ways to fail</u> *but only a few ways to succeed.* That is dead on correct!

It should be obvious that perfecting technique in any of the lifts takes a lot of work, and constant practice. Mastering technique takes time and there is no short cut. But if you wanted something easy, you would be playing fantasy football, not trying to lift big iron.

Think about your lifting technique as being as complex as a golf swing or as complex as diving off a 10-meter platform. You can master the fundamentals, but you always need to insure that small bad habits don't creep in. You need regular feedback on what you are doing that is right and what might be wrong.

A good coach will be able to help you make the small changes that can make a huge difference in your performance. It is the small things that a good coach will see that are completely invisible to the novice.

Doing the small things right is critical to peak performance. That is why the pro golfers have coaches helping them with their swing and the best basketball players have coaches to help them with their shooting.

For this reason, I suggest that as you get better and better, it is important that you find a good powerlifting coach. This is a person who has trained many successful powerlifters. A good coach is going to see small subtle things that you need to correct.

When you are just starting out, you can use this book as a guide to developing your technique. Once you get to be more experienced, you will want to find someone who really knows the sport of powerlifting.

I keep harping on the fact that 99% of the "personal trainers" around have no idea how to coach powerlifting. I say this from having known hundreds of them. All are excellent at helping total novices get involved with "exercise". After that, the good trainers will have some sport or activity that they really know well. For the vast majority it is something other than powerlifting.

Another thing that will help you become the best you can be, is to train with other competitive lifters. The community of likeminded people can do a huge amount to improve your performance. They can coach you and encourage you in ways that no one else can.

There is a good chance that these lifters will not train at your gym. But, it will help if you can find out where they are training, and arrange to work out with them on some occasions.

Generally, there will be a small group of competitive lifters in any community of any size. I have even found a powerlifting gym in a tiny town (Gordon, Nebraska).

In the section on competing in powerlifting I'll show you how to find lifters and coaches in your area.

Contest Legal Bench Press Equipment

Shortly I'll get into the training cycles for the bench press. However, before doing that I believe it is really important to discuss bench press equipment, since it has such a major impact on your ability to train effectively.

I'm assuming that most of you will be training without bench press support shirts as they are extremely difficult to use and impossible to get on and off by yourself. If you are using them, you are probably training with a group of powerlifters.

The majority of you will be training "raw" or without support equipment. This is what I recommend if you are in your first two to three years of powerlifting. For most of you, it will be the only way you ever train or compete.

However, the equipment issues I need to address at the start of this section apply to the bench you use and the bars you use. Those issues apply to everyone.

I'll discuss the personal equipment (shirts and wraps) after that.

Bench Press Equipment

There are two types of equipment you need to consider when training for a competition bench press. The first is the bench and the lifting bar. The second personal equipment you may want to use.

Competition benches and bars

Let's begin with what constitutes a legal competition bench.

The bench you will use in a contest will conform to all the rules. The bench you find in your local gym may have a design that is totally out of line with the rules.

The most common problem with gym benches is that they are not of legal height. The bench should be between 17-17 ½ inches high (42-45 cm). This measurement is from the floor to the top of the pad. A lot of benches in gyms are lower than this and a few are higher.

The width of the bench must be 11.5 to 12.5 inches (29-32 cm). Usually gym benches are within this dimension.

The height of the bench is important because it determines how you plant your feet when you set up. If you are of average height or above, benches that are lower than competition standards make it very hard to get tight, and assume proper position on the bench.

Gym benches are typically padded in ways that competition benches are not. Padding can create some instability if it is too thick. This is the last thing you want if you are holding a heavy weight at arm's length.

The upright stands that hold the barbell must be vertical in a competition bench. Gym benches often have the weight rack at an angle. This can create problems for getting the bar in and out of the rack. Vertical rack stands allow you to take the weight off the rack in the optima position for a strong press, and minimize the chance that you might hit the rack during the upward press movement.

You should have a tape measure in your workout bag to check the dimensions of benches you may use in the gym. Sometimes you have no option but to use nonstandard equipment in training. It can be a big help to know the difference between the equipment you use for training and the bench equipment you will see in a meet.

The bench press bar is another piece of equipment you need to know.

All competition bars will have an area between the collars of roughly 52 inches (131 cm). Approximately 9.6 inches (24.5 cm) from each collar is a machined marking, usually a clear space in the knurling a few centimeters wide. This mark defines the maximum hand spacing width any lifter can use in competition.

The rule states that if a lifter uses a wide grip, the mark must be covered by the lifters hand. This means you can place your hands on the outside of the mark, just so long as the mark is fully covered when you wrap your hand around the bar.

The legal distance between the two marks is roughly 32 inches (81 cm).

You can take a narrower grip if you wish, but you cannot take a wider grip than that shown by the markings on the bar.

Now a word of caution about the lifting bars normally used in fitness gyms. The markings on the bar may bear no relationship to the marks required for powerlifting. There may be markings on the bar, but I have found that they are often nothing other than random decoration.

If you train in a regular fitness gym, you need to take your own tape measure and carefully mark the bar you use. The mark should be one you can see when you are lying on your back positioning your hands for the lift. Marking pen is often a good choice.

If you train with regulation powerlifting bars, there should be no problem. However, it is best to check. Finding out you have been training using an illegal grip width can cause you a lot of grief.

Now let's take a brief look at personal support equipment.

Support gear: shirts, wraps and lifting belts

In the quarter century I competed, I saw a dramatic evolution of support equipment for the bench press. Back in the 1980's the bench shirts were simple, and relatively cheap. Even then they could add a lot to your bench press.

Over the past two decades the technology and design of bench shirts has dramatically increased their effectiveness. Some large men have benched 800-1000 pounds while wearing specialized bench shirts.

At the same time, the impact of the shirts on the amount someone could lift has been so great that major national lifting associations have begun separate competitions for unequipped lifters (no support gear) and equipped lifters. The unequipped lifting is called "raw" lifting.

Raw lifters compete wearing a non-supportive singlet and a t-shirt. Equipped lifters compete wearing shirts that are approved by the individual lifting associations.

I have competed both raw and in support gear. The support gear makes a dramatic difference in how much I can bench and squat. However, for a number of reasons, I have directed this book at people who will train without support equipment. There are multiple reasons for this.

The first is that all of the shirts are *extremely difficult to use.* The only way I would ever suggest that someone buy and try to use a shirt is if they are working with a *very experienced* powerlifting coach who knows how to get the shirts to perform for the lifter.

When I say an "experienced" powerlifting coach, I mean someone who has many lifters competing on a regular basis using bench shirts. Some personal trainer who "has seen one on the internet" will not be able to help you much, and may put you in considerable danger.

I strongly suggest that you not use bench support gear unless you can train with a highly knowledgeable coach and a group of lifters who use the shirts most of the time. This is for the following reasons:

First, on your own, you will have a limited idea of what shirt to buy, and they are very expensive (as in $150-$300+). There are lots of choices, and shirt technology and rules governing their use change regularly. The only people who will be up to date on this information will be those who compete regularly, and know what shirts are legal in which associations.

Second, you cannot get into a shirt by yourself, and you cannot get out of a shirt by yourself. It takes 1-3 other people to get you into the shirt, depending on your size and how tight it fits. If you are going to get *any* benefit from a shirt, it has to be *extremely tight!*

How tight? If the shirt fits properly, your arms will be suspended parallel to the floor, and you will not be able to touch your lifting belt.

Because the shirt has to fit very tight to give you any benefit, getting the shirt on you correctly is something only a few users know how to do. There may be some videos on You Tube, but people who regularly use the shirts are the only ones who know how to make them fit correctly.

Correct fit will include such things as seeing that the sleeves are rotated properly, the neck hole does not drift upward, the sides are pulled down and that the front is pulled down and secured by your lifting belt before you lie down on the bench. None of this can be done by someone who has not regularly used the shirt.

Oh….when you are on the bench doing a bench press in a shirt, it is *very painful!* The shirt will constrict you in ways you never thought possible. That is why it works! It takes a huge amount of the weight load.

Using shirts can be extremely dangerous if you don't have experienced spotters. Because the weights you will be using are immense compared to what you could do raw, and the fit of the shirt is critical to give you any boost, you have a high likelihood of losing control of a big weight when it is either descending to your chest, or partway up.

Most shirts will force your arms up toward your face. To get benefit from the shirt, you literally "fight" the shirt by forcing the weight into the area of greatest resistance. If you lose control of the bar, it can flip back into your face, or land on your neck. The only thing that will save you from serious injury or death is a good spotter or group of spotters.

When I trained with a group of lifters who used bench shirts, regardless of the weight on the bar, we had a spotter at each end of the bar, and one in the middle. When the big guys were lifting, we had *really* big guys spotting. If someone lost control of a weight, it landed in some big hands instantly. No one ever got hurt, but only because everyone knew how to spot, and we always insured that spotters could control the weight if the lifter dropped it.

Spotting a big bench press when wearing a bench shirt is nothing that you should ever leave to a couple dudes you round up in the gym. The guy who is spotting in the middle should be able to deadlift the weight, and the two on the ends should be able to be able to manage a few hundred pounds suddenly dropped into their hands.

In short, if you want to lift equipped, in my opinion it is mandatory that you do so with a group of people who are really skilled at using bench shirts. You may have to hunt around your area to find where these people train, but in most cities you can usually find them.

Otherwise, train raw and compete raw.

Before I leave the subject of personal support equipment, let me address wrist wraps.

Wrist protection wraps are legal for both raw and equipped lifting. They can be useful for protecting your wrists while supporting really heavy weights. High quality wrist wraps are not particularly expensive, and I suggest that every lifter have one pair for use in the bench press and the squat.

Wrist wraps come in different lengths ranging from longer ones (2' or 60 cm) that will go around your wrist several times, to mid lengths (around 20" or 50 cm) that will do two or three turns around the wrist. They have a thumb hook on one end, and a Velcro fastener on the other. They are very easy to put on and take off.

The wraps are elastic, and there is a real advantage to wrapping them tight for heavier lifts.

You should be aware that during competition, no part of the wrap can touch the lifting bar. This includes the thumb hook which is easy to take off once the wrap is in place.

You can find a source for the best in wraps and other lifting equipment on my site at www.MidLifeHardBody.com

You want to have a high quality lifting belt to use for all three lifts. The only ones worth spending your money on are those that are contest legal. As I noted elsewhere, these belts are never sold in sporting goods stores. They are available only from suppliers who specialize in powerlifting gear. See my site www.MidLifeHardBody.com for good sources.

A lifting belt is another piece of equipment that is critical for bench pressing. Belts are legal for both raw and equipped lifting.

As noted earlier, you will be pressing your abs hard against the belt during the bench press. This is critical for generating the most force you can during the lift. That happens whether you are lifting raw, or lifting with a support shirt.

If you are lifting with a supportive shirt, the tightened belt will keep the shirt in place during your lift.

For raw lifting all you need is a belt and wrist wraps.

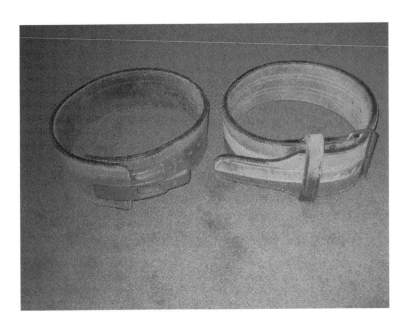

Lever Belt and Buckle Style Belt

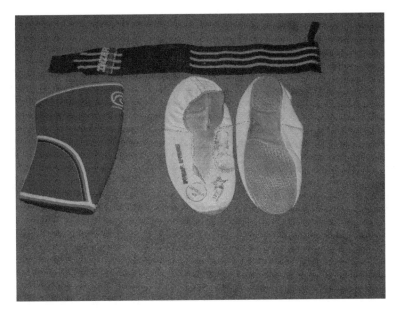

Wrist wrap, knee sleeve, and deadlifting slippers

Chapter 8

Bench Press Training Cycles

In the next section, I'll show you five different training cycles for the bench press. Each one will include a specific amount of bench pressing and then assistance exercises to be done immediately after doing the bench press sets.

Each cycle will be done for a maximum of eight weeks. After eight weeks, change your program.

The bench pressing and assistance work will be done **one day per week.** This is called "heavy day" in powerlifters jargon.

In all of the powerlifting training program you will have one heavy day each week for the squat, bench press and deadlift. You will also have a "light day" when you will do a series of exercises that include support work for all three lifts.

During each week you will have **three days of recovery.** It is particularly critical that people over age 50 observe these recovery days if you want to improve your strength and power.

With that introduction, let's now proceed to the five bench press training cycles:

1. Foundation Cycle
2. Explosive Strength Cycle
3. Builder/Power Cage Cycle
4. Explosive Power II
5. Contest Peaking Cycle

Bench Press Cycle #1 - Foundation Cycle

With this program you build foundation strength for the bench press. Begin your bench press training here. The cool thing is you can use this program over and over again to enhance your power.

The foundation program is 4 sets of 5 reps of the bench press, peaking on the 3rd set. It's common for younger lifters to do 5 sets of 5 reps, but, I believe that the maximum benefit for a lifter over age 50 will come in the first four sets. The fifth set will only serve to add to fatigue.

The weight you use to start this cycle will be a percentage of your one rep maximum. Below, I list the percentage of one rep max you should use for this cycle:

Set 1: 65%

Set 2: 75%

Set 3: 80%

Set 4: 75%

Every two weeks increase the weights you use by 5 pounds (2.5Kg). If all the weights in a set feel light, you can increase the weight once a week. You will be on this program for eight weeks, so the total increase in the weights you are using will be at least 20-25 pounds (10 Kg).

You should use perfect form on all reps, and do a long pause on the first two reps of each set. You can do a shorter pause on the last three. In no case should you do a "touch and go" rep. If you have to do a touch and go to make the rep, the weight is too heavy.

Twenty repetitions of the bench is a considerable amount of work. You will be doing two workouts a week, and the total number of reps you will do over the cycle is 320. This is a big volume of work, as you will be doing assistance exercises as well as regular bench presses.

Assistance Exercises

The assistance exercises for the foundation program emphasize building pressing strength as well as developing the support muscles in the triceps and lats to help push and stabilize the lift.

Standing Barbell Press

The standing press is an excellent way to develop overall body strength and superior pressing power. It is a greatly undervalued lift these days, but will pay you huge dividends over the long haul.

You will do this movement for 3 sets of 5 reps. Increase the weight on the second set.

In all the assistance exercises, select a weight that you can do easily for the first four reps with modest exertion on the final rep. Starting too heavy will cause your progress to quickly plateau. You will need to experiment to find the proper starting weight in your first session.

Over the course of eight weeks, you can increase the weight when you can do five reps easily.

Begin by loading the barbell while it sits on the floor. <u>Never ever</u> take the bar off a squat rack to do presses. Only Ken and Barbie do it that way.

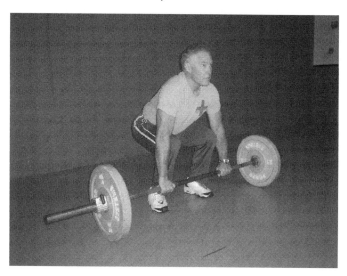

Bring the bar to your shoulders (power clean) with a grip slightly wider than your shoulders. Lock your legs, feet, buttocks, back, abs and neck. Your entire body should be tight. At that point take a deep breath and hold it. Push the weight up using every muscle you can recruit, but without moving anything but your arms.

Once the bar is moving off your shoulders push it forward just enough to clear your nose. Once the weight is past your nose, continue the press by pushing the bar slightly backward so that you drive it up to the lockout over the top of your head.

When the bar is locked out overhead, release your breath and lower the bar to your shoulders for the next rep. Take another deep breath and repeat the lift.

You should NEVER do a "push press" lift where you bend your knees and jerk the weight upward. That is a terrific lift, but it is completely different from what you need to be doing here.

The standing press is a difficult lift and one reason it is rarely practiced any more is because it is so difficult. As I said, you will get big benefits from practicing this lift correctly.

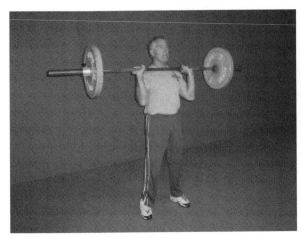
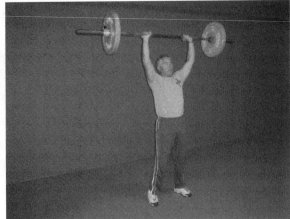

Barbell Rowing

The lats contribute a huge amount of power for your bench press, and it is important that you develop their strength along with your pecs, deltoids and triceps.

You will do 4 sets of 5 reps in this movement. You can increase the weight on the 2nd and 3rd sets if you wish.

The barbell row is one of the movements that will give you a lot of power through the range of motion that you want to develop for a big bench press.

Begin with the barbell on the floor. Take a grip that is the same as the hand spacing you use in the bench press. Keeping your body bent over so that your trunk is parallel to the floor, take a deep breath, tighten your body and pull the weight up to your *waist*. Do not pull it to your chest.

Keep your back flat, your abs locked down tight, and your head erect.

Release your breath, and lower the weight to the starting position. Take another deep breath and repeat the movement.

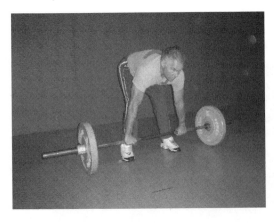
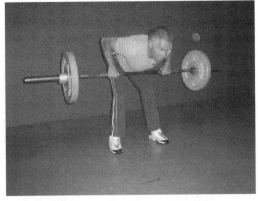

Dumbbell Triceps Press

The final assistance movement in this program is the dumbbell triceps press. The purpose of this movement is to strengthen the triceps through a full range of motion. You should always stretch the triceps fully at the bottom of this lift. Don't cheat and use a heavier weight by limiting how far down you lower the weight.

You will do this movement for 2 sets of 8 reps. The weight should be relatively light because the aim is to extend the triceps through a full range of motion.

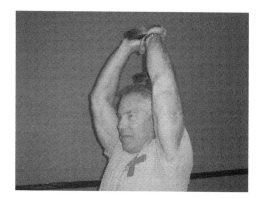 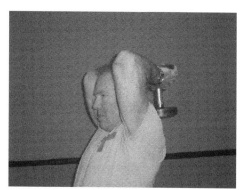

Note: The gentleman in the photographs is my friend Ed. At age 65 he is a practicing attorney, and both massively strong, and very athletic. He benches over 300 at a bodyweight of 180 and is a top notch downhill skier. Just for fun, he works in mountain rescue.

Bench Press Cycle #2 - Explosive Strength Cycle

The explosive strength cycle is designed to maximize the burst of power you get off the chest. The emphasis will be on doing perfect reps, and pushing the bench press upward with as much force as you can manage.

Because the emphasis will be on generating maximum force, the number of reps in each set will be strictly limited to 2. No matter how good you feel, keep the reps to 2 on all 5 sets.

Take the weight off the rack and hold it at arm's length. Lower the weight to your chest using perfect technique. When on the chest hold the weight for a count of 3, then drive it upward with all the force you can mobilize.

Begin your sets using a weight that is relatively easy for you to manage on both reps. You will increase the weight each set until you find it mildly difficult to push the second rep. When you reach that weight, decrease the weight on the next set.

I recommend that you experiment with the weight you use, and start with something around 60% of your 1 current rep maximum. It is important that you not go too heavy on these sets since you are training your central nervous system to put out maximum force. You will be surprised at how quickly you can burn out if you work too heavy.

As always, practice perfect technique on all bench presses. When the weights get heavy is when most people begin to see their form deteriorate.

You should stay on this program for four weeks.

Assistance Exercises

The assistance work on the explosive strength portion of the program will be aimed at building stabilizing muscles and enhancing triceps strength. The high stress of the explosive bench presses will give your body plenty to adapt to. The strength building assistance work will seem a little bit like a break.

Standing Dumbbell Press

The standing dumbbell press will build balanced power in both shoulders and work the stabilizer muscles as well.

Select dumbbells that you can manage relatively well for five reps. You may increase the weight only once during the month you are on this program. That is fine, since you are training on this lift for stability and to insure equal strength from each arm.

Begin with the dumbbells on the floor. Clean them to your shoulders and hold them with your palms facing inward.

Take a deep breath, tense your entire body and push *both* the dumbbells upward so that the movement is straight up then slightly back when they pass the top of your head. The goal is to drive them into the stable groove where you have the greatest strength.

You can release your breath when the press is locked out overhead. Lower the dumbbells to your shoulders and repeat again.

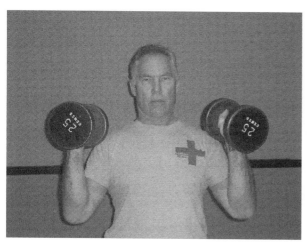
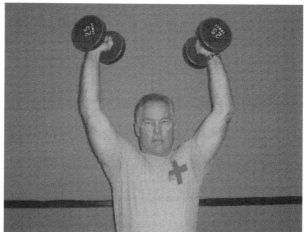

You should do 4 sets of 5 reps of this exercise.

One Arm Rowing

The dumbbell row movement works your back, arms and neck. All of these are crucial for building a big bench.

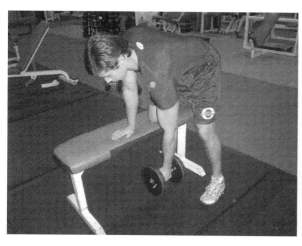
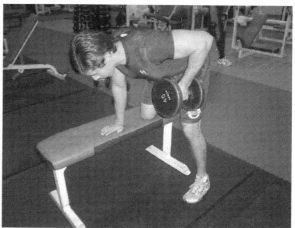

You will be doing 5 reps with each arm to make one set. Do a total of 4 sets of 5 reps on each side.

Put a dumbbell on the floor, and bend over at the waist so that your trunk is parallel to the floor. For the first set, grab the dumbbell in your right hand, and place your left hand on your left knee for stability. You can also kneel on a flat bench as shown in the picture. Keep a flat back throughout. Keep your head erect and looking forward.

Take a deep breath and pull the dumbbell up to your waist. Don't pull it to your chest. Release your breath and lower the weight to the starting position. Repeat five times with each hand for one set.

"Skull Crusher"

This is one of those exercises you will love to hate. The "skull crusher" is one of the great movements for building really powerful triceps.

You will be grinding out 4 sets of 5 reps with this exercise. The big benefit comes from doing this with perfect technique and not cheating….so don't cheat.

Ideally you can use a short barbell for this exercise. A longer barbell becomes difficult to control, since you will be using a narrow grip.

Set the barbell on the floor at the end of a flat bench. Sit on the end of the bench, and pick up the barbell so that it is resting in your lap. You should grasp the bar with a narrow grip, with 8"-12" between your hands. Lie back on the bench and adjust the barbell so that you can press it to arm's length over your chest.

When the bar is over your chest, take a deep breath, tense your body, and keeping your elbows pointed at the ceiling, lower the weight to your forehead.

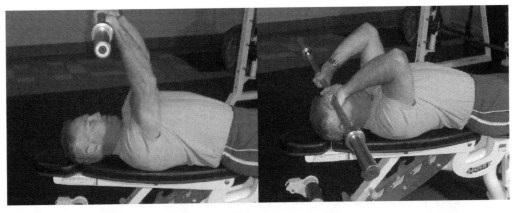

Keep your elbows pointed at the ceiling and raise the bar up to the starting position. All the work should be done by your triceps.

The heavy work in this program is in the explosive bench presses. One month of explosive training will be enough to propel you to bigger heights.

It is important to remember that no program works for very long, and this particular program is one that will only help you for about a month. These "mini-cycles" are an integral part of what the great Louie Simmons calls "conjugate training". This is used by VERY advanced lifters.

Bench Press Cycle #3 – Builder/Power Cage Training

This is a cycle that will really push you, as you will be doing regular bench presses, and adding heavy overloads in the power cage. When you do this you should stay on it no longer than eight weeks. You can do it for a shorter time if you desire.

Whenever you are doing serious heavy lifting, you should be particularly aware of the chances for injury or aggravation to your joints and muscles. Older lifters can be particularly vulnerable if they have some accumulated damage to shoulders, back or neck. For that reason, I repeat over and over that if you are worried about getting hurt, your intuition is probably correct.

If you strain something or "tweak" an old injury during a workout, immediately stop heavy lifting. It is possible to build up mind-blowing strength, but not if you are regularly injured. It is really important that you not try to "train your way through pain". For those of us who are senior lions, learning when to take a day off, quit a workout, or change up what we are doing is the difference between having a long healthy career as a fit person, or being hobbled by chronic injuries.

Backing off when your body tells you it is time to go easy is the essence of training smart!

With that caveat, let's look at the builder/power cage cycle.

You start with doing the regular bench press for 5 sets of 2 reps, with the heaviest weight being used on the 3rd set. The recommended starting weights for this cycle are:

Set 1: 65% of current 1 rep max

Set 2: 75% of current 1 rep max

Set 3: 85% of current 1 rep max

Set 4: 75% of current 1 rep max

Set 5; 65% of current 1 rep max

You should increase the weights 5 lbs every two weeks.

As before, move briskly through the workout sets. Take no more than three minutes between sets.

It always bears repeating that perfect technique is required on all lifts. Doing lifts badly will only retard progress.

Assistance Work

  Power Cage Lock Outs

The power cage offers an opportunity to train "part" of the lift with much heavier weights than could be done when doing full range movements. This is done by setting the weighted bar on the support pins at different heights off the chest.

When the weight is in position, set up on the bench under the bar, get tight, and push the weight to arm's length in a full lock out.

There are three main positions to use in the power cage. The first is at the sticking point a few inches off the chest, the second is when the bar is 4-6 inches below full lock out and the third is an inch or so below full lockout.

Working at the sticking point can be very useful for training to exert maximum force at a point in the lift where things often "go south". It can also help you "feel" what might be taking place that cause problems in the full lift.

The first point to set the support bars is so that the bar sits about 2-3" (5-8 cm) off your chest when you are lying on your back on a flat bench. Load the bar to 10% less than your 1 rep max. Adjust your body on the bench so that the bar is positioned exactly as it would be if you were doing a full bench press.

At that point, take a deep breath, get completely tight, and push the bar up to a full lockout.

The first time you try this you may find that you are really weak at this point in the lift. You may have to lower the weight to successfully move it from a dead stop. That is the purpose of this lift, to correct weak points in your bench press.

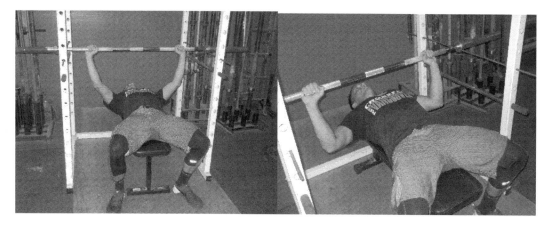

Upper Lock out position   **Lower Lock out position**

The second point where you move the bar from a dead stop will be when your arms are almost fully extended. That will be 4-6" (10-15 cm) from full lock out.

The third position is 1-2" below full lock out (3-5 cm). When you lift the bar from a dead stop at this position, you will be able to move a huge amount of weight. The advantage of doing this will be that not only will it help your lockout; it will make your regular bench press feel lighter.

As explained earlier, the static contraction of your muscles in this exercise will make you stronger through all ranges of motion.

In both of these lifts in the power cage, you should only do single repetitions. In total, do no more than nine individual lifts in total. These lifts really stress your central nervous system, and you can burn out quickly.

Caveat: If you train with knowledgeable lifting partners, there is an advantage to doing partial lifts placing wooden blocks on the chest and controlling the bar through the lift. However, this takes one spotter to hold the wood block on your chest, and at least one spotter behind the bench to rescue you if the lift fails. You must have spotters or this becomes very dangerous.

I'll talk more about using boards for partial lifts in the section on advanced bench press training below.

You should always use the cage for the most extreme heavy lock outs. This is because you will be using weights that may be too much for one spotter to help you control.

Incline Dumbbell Presses

Using dumbbells on the incline bench trains the shoulder and pecs while forcing you to control the weights in each hand separately. This is great for activating all the muscles needed to stabilize the weight.

Begin with weights that allow you to do five reps, but not easily. Your objective will be to increase the weight of the dumbbells you use over the course of the eight-week cycle. To do this you can't begin with a weight that is right at your limit, or you will plateau quickly. So, select a weight that will allow you to progress, but not train at your limit.

As noted earlier, most incline benches in gyms are fabricated with so that the incline is permanently at 45 degrees. If by chance your incline bench is adjustable, set it for a 45-degree incline rather than a setting closer to vertical.

You will be doing 3 sets of 5 reps.

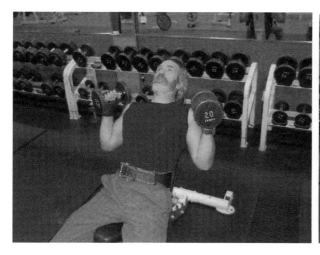 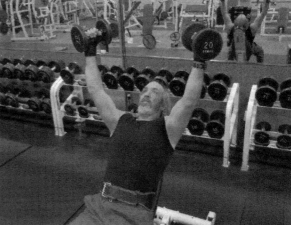

Starting Position   **Lock out position**

Begin by cleaning the dumbbells to your shoulders. Then sit down on the bench. Lie back into the starting positon and insure your feet are firmly planted on the floor.

Take a deep breath and hold it. Get your body tight as you should be doing for every lift. Dig your feet into the floor, tighten your abs, and press the dumbbells overhead. You can exhale when the weights are locked out at arm's length.

Lower the weight under control to your shoulders and repeat until you have done five reps. Then with the weights on your shoulders, stand up and lower the weights to your thighs. At that point, put them on the floor for your next set, or back in the dumbbell rack when you have finished.

Close Grip Bench Press

Close grip bench press is one of the great triceps movements that will really help your bench press.

Lie on a bench press bench and take a relatively narrow grip on the bar as shown below. The spacing between the hands can be anywhere from 8" (21 cm) to 12" (30 cm) or slightly wider. The purpose of the narrow grip is to force all of the effort of the lift on to your triceps.

Lift the bar off the rack and hold it at arm's length. Take a deep breath and hold it. Be tight as usual. Lower the bar under control to your chest. Pause briefly and push it back to arm's length.

You will be doing 3 sets of 5 reps on this.

Select a weight that is somewhat demanding on the final rep of the first set. Make a small increase in the weight on the second set and the third set.

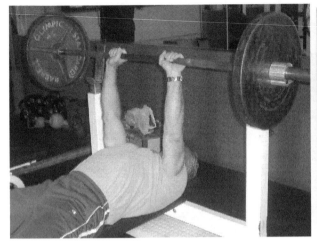
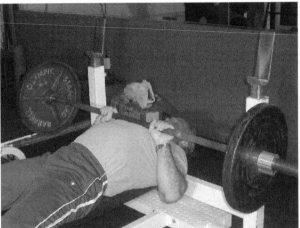

Starting position   **Bottom position**

Upright Rowing

Upright rowing is designed to build the rear deltoids, your upper back and neck all of which are critical to having a big bench press.

You will be doing 3 sets of 5 reps.

Load the barbell and place it on the floor. Take a grip where your hands are 6" (15 cm) to 12" (30 cm) apart. Stand erect with the barbell in your hands.

Tighten your body, take a deep breath, flex your abs, crush the bar with your grip and lift the weight deliberately up the front of your torso to shoulder height by flaring your elbows out and up. Keep your hands close to your body. Do not bend over and heave the bar upward. The lift should be relatively slow and smooth.

This is not a narrow grip power clean. The bar should be lifted slowly rather than quickly. It should take about a full second for you to move the weight from the start position to the finish position.

Lower the bar under control to the starting position and repeat for five reps.

You should make small increases in the weight after each set.

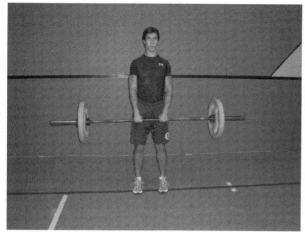
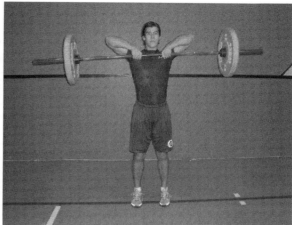

Starting position **Top of the pull**

The builder program will get your baseload strength to a superior level. It should also correct any weak spots in your bench press.

When you have done this program for eight weeks, you will can go to the peaking routine to prepare for a competition, or change to one of the other programs. In any event, eight weeks is the longest time you should do the builder program.

Bench Press Cycle #4 - Explosive Strength II

This is another "mini-cycle" so you will only train on this for a month before changing to another bench press routine.

A different approach to training explosiveness on the bench press is to use very light weights (50% of current 1 rep max) and emphasize moving the bar as fast as humanly possible during the lift.

As noted, the heaviest weight used in the bench press portion of this program is 50% of your current 1 rep maximum. This should be your current 1 rep max, not the "best you could do in college".

The purpose is to train the central nervous system to put out maximum force. Over time it has been determined that lifters tend to train themselves to put out less than maximum force, particularly if they train with high repetitions. For this reason, Louie Simmons devised the "speed program", 7 sets of 2 reps at 50% of maximum.

Each rep should be done with perfect technique, and with as much acceleration as you can possibly place on the bar. Pause each rep on the chest for a count of 2 and then explode the bar upward as rapidly as you can move it.

One major difference between other routines and this one is that you will take only *30 seconds* between sets. That means you should finish your 7 sets of 2 reps in well under 10 minutes.

Even though your bench press training was light, the assistance work will be the heavy part of your workout. You should push yourself on the assistance work.

Even though the weights will be heavy, you should keep the pace of the training brisk. Keep your recovery time between dumbbell presses to 3 minutes or less, stay at 2 minutes for the lat pull downs, and roughly the same for incline presses.

Assistance Training

Dumbbell Bench Press

Dumbbell bench presses are one of the more dangerous movements routinely done in the gym. The lift itself is not dangerous, but the way many lifters get on and off the bench is really dangerous.

If you have been training around any group of lifters who work with dumbbells on a bench, there always seem to be a group who simply drop the weights on the floor when they are finished with a set. This results in an impressive sound, and can create a bit of a problem for anyone in the immediate vicinity of the bench.

Although it sounds really macho, and draws all kinds of attention, dropping weights puts the lifters shoulders at significant risk. Once a lifter relaxes and lets the weights fall, he has no control over where they go. Injuries from this practice almost never happen, but when they do, they are usually catastrophic.

I recall one accident where a lifter dropped the weights at the end of a set, and one dumbbell descended to the floor with no problem, but somehow he didn't release both dumbbells at the same time and one dumbbell got stuck in his hand. This pulled his shoulder joint out of the socket. Lots of really bad pain, followed by surgery. He was able to comb his hair with that arm about a year later.

The point is, don't ever risk your bod needlessly. There are safe ways to get on and off a flat bench while holding big dumbbells. In fact, I'll be telling your how right now.

First of all, grasp the dumbbells so that when you sit down on the end of the bench, you can put the dumbbells on your lap. Once they are steady on your lap, you can lie back on the bench and adjust the dumbbells up to your chest. At this point you are ready to do a dumbbell press.

The highest risk comes when you have finished your presses. Instead of allowing the dumbbells to free fall to the floor, you should hold them on your chest, and slide them down your torso until they rest on your legs. At that point, sit up. The dumbbells will be on your lap, and fully under your control. At that point, you can stand up and put the dumbbells on the floor.

If this sounds simple, it is. It may be simple, but it can save you from a massive injury.

Now….on to the dumbbell bench press. You will be doing 5 sets of 5-4-3-2-5 reps.

On the first set, select a weight that you can manage reasonably for a set of 5 reps.

On the second set, increase the weight by 5 pounds, and do 4 reps. Increase the weight again on the third set. Continue to increase until you do 2 reps on the 4th set. Return to your starting weight for the 5th set and do 5 reps.

On successive workouts try to do 1 more rep with the weight you could only manage 4 with previously. When you can do 5 reps, increase the weight and drop back to 3 or 4 reps.

The idea is to try to increase by at least 1 rep on 1 of the sets each workout. If you can increase on 2 sets, that is OK too. The basic idea is to *gradually* build up your strength so that you are lifting heavier weights than you were when you began.

This is a lot of work volume, so don't try to improve more than 1 rep on 2 sets each workout. If you keep your increases modest, they will be steady. Push too much too soon, and your progress will stop.

As on all pressing movements, before your press, you want to have your entire body as tight as possible in order to put out the maximum force during the lift. You will be starting the lift on the chest, so you inhale forcefully and hold it while the weights are on your chest.

Your elbows can be either tight against your body, or flared out. This will depend on your past history of shoulder injuries, or how you prefer to bench press. I found that after the first ten years of powerlifting, I kept my elbows in against my sides as my right shoulder gradually developed a problem.

Because you are using dumbbells, you will be pressing the weights with a narrow grip. This will force a lot of the work onto your triceps. Because each arm is working independently, the movement will also activate stabilizer muscles.

When working with heavy weights, it is usually advisable to enlist the help of a spotter. I have discussed this with regard to the squat and bench press. It is also a good idea to use a spotter with the dumbbell bench press. But, you need to train them to do exactly what you want, or they can cause you more problems than they alleviate.

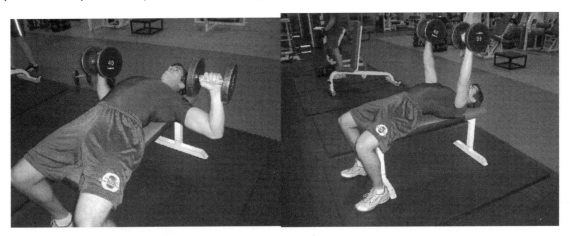

Starting position **Lockout position**

The first thing the spotter needs to know is that if you can't make a lift, where do you want the weight to go. In the dumbbell bench press, the safest place for the dumbbell to come to rest is on your chest. If you can't make the lift, your spotter should help you stabilize the weight at the starting point of the lift.

At that point, you can slide the weight down to your lap and sit up, or you can ask the spotter to lift them off of you (at the same time). After you have just missed a heavy lift is not the time to think about dropping weights on the floor.

Lat Pull Down

The lat pull down can be a major contributor to the power of your push off the chest. As you recall, the first drive out of the bottom of the bench press comes from the lats.

This is a popular body building movement, and one of the very few machine movements that I recommend. It is very much like a chin up, and because you are able to change the weight you pull, it is possible to build up a really powerful lat pull.

For power training, you will be doing five sets of five reps. You should select a weight that is as heavy as you can manage for five reps. Pull the bar down and touch the top of your chest on each rep.

As you move through your sets, you can increase the weight so that you can only grind out 2 or 3 reps. Just try to do more reps on that weight the next time you work out.

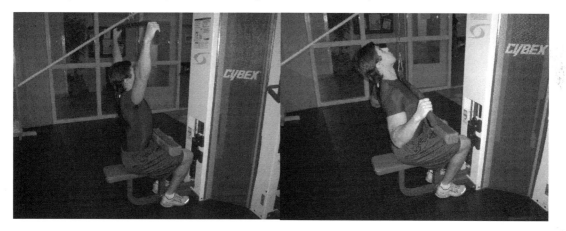

Starting pull down   **Pull the bar to your chest**

One word of caution. You should always do your heavy pull downs bringing the bar *in front* of your face, and never behind the neck. The movement behind the neck puts extraordinary strain on the shoulder joint and can quickly lead to a nagging injury.

You should move the weight by pulling down with your arm and back muscles. You should NOT do the movement by hanging on to the bar, then leaning way back to pull the weight stack up, and then quickly moving forward to touch the bar to your chest. That is lame! It also does not do you much good.

Incline Bench Press

The incline bench press makes you push hard from a slightly different angle. This can lead to some awesome power.

After doing high speed bench presses and heavy dumbbell work, you should not go all out on the incline, but keep it to weights that you can manage with "some" work for five reps. Don't go for broke here.

The incline bench press works the upper part of your chest as well as the triceps, and shoulders. All contribute to a big bench.

At the end of your bench training session, aim for 3 sets of 5 reps. Increase the weight on the second set, and decrease it on the third.

Load the bar on the support racks and then get on the bench. Take the same grip you would use in your bench press and lift the bar off the rack.

You will begin this exercise with your arms extended overhead. Take a deep breath and bring the weight down to your chest. Your elbows will be in against your sides when you lower the weight.

As always, make your entire body tight, and recruit as much strength as you can. Try to bend the bar, crush the bar with your grip, pause the weight briefly on your chest and push it back to arm's length. You exhale when your arms are fully extended.

Take no more than two minutes between sets.

Bench Press Cycle #5 - Contest Peaking Program

When you are preparing for a competition you will do a peaking routing to improve your personal best for each lift. You will be doing all of the peaking routines at the same time, assuming that you are going to compete in all three lifts.

The bottom line goal of doing these routines is to have a great contest and do your best lifting. This means that you are going to have to exercise good sense and discipline and not over train or spend too much energy working out. The point is to do great in the contest, *not leave your best lifts in the gym!*

The late basketball great Wilt Chamberlin is alleged to have said something like "you want to win the *game*, not the workout". I mention this because there is a tendency among gym rats and power trainees to constantly push for more weight and more reps in a workout. This tendency to work like an animal can really work against you when you are trying to prepare to do your best lifts.

It is essential to remember that even though you may feel like Superman, being over 50 imposes some limits on how fast you can recover. It is best to work within those limitations. Get lots of sleep and if you are tired, cut back on training. You will discover that by "training smart" you can obliterate a lot of your old personal bests.

Throughout this book I have made reference to sticking to a plan, not over training and recovering between training sessions. Nowhere is that more important than when you are trying to peak for a competitive event.

As I'll remind you again and again, during a peaking program (as well as others) recovery and rest are of equal importance (perhaps more) than what you do in the gym.

The great Louie Simmons once said "there is nothing you can do to get stronger in the final week before a contest. However, there is *a lot you can do to get weaker!!!*"

Now…after competing for a quarter of a century, I can assure you that at various times in my lifting career, I was certain that the "rules don't apply to me". I was prone to do "one more set, or an extra workout, etc." I always did my best lifting when rested. Hopefully you can learn from some of my mistakes.

Anatomy of a peaking routine.

Peaking is going to be somewhat different than the other training cycles since as you go through it, you will gradually scale back the amount of work you do, and really focus on getting prepared for doing a single rep at your maximum capability.

There is a basic structure to all peaking routines that I discussed earlier, but bears repeating again. You begin a multi-week cycle by doing ONE workout per week on each lift where you exert major effort on one of the three competitive lifts. For example, the program shown below would be for "bench press day".

On the day when you concentrate on the bench press, you will focus on putting the bulk of your effort into a small number of low repetition sets. You begin the cycle by working with weights well below your 1 rep maximum, and over the cycle you increase the weight, and reduce the number of sets and reps. Just before the contest you have primed yourself to do your best possible single.

When you prepare for a peaking routine, you begin by working backward from the lift you plan to do in a contest. Let's say that at present your best bench press is 300 pounds and your goal for the contest is 315. You would prepare your peaking plan by starting at the date of the contest with a lift of 315, and working backward to the present using percentages of this lift to calculate what you needed to do in each workout leading up to the contest.

Now, how far back do you go for a peaking routine? I suggest that you do a peaking routine for no longer than eight weeks and no less than six weeks.

I arrived at this range mainly from my own and other lifting friends experience. In the old days, some of the guru's used to design twelve week peaking routines. When I followed this advice, I found that I was always at my best with four to six weeks to go before the meet. Thus, I suggest that peaking routines be shorter.

Let's go back to the desired 315 bench press and see how to plan backward from that goal.

You will do your bench press peaking routine once a week. On you "light" day, you will do light (50% of max) bench work and some light assistance work). The light day work will taper off over the eight-week cycle.

Here is a sample eight-week program for "heavy day" to increase the contest bench press from 300 to 315.

All of the weights are based on calculating a percentage of the current one rep max.

Contest day: Planned attempts in the bench press: 280-305-315

One week out: Single rep at 305

Two weeks out: Single reps at 290 and 300

Three weeks out: Double at 260   Single at 285

Four weeks out: Double at 245, Double at 255

Five weeks out: Triple at 225, Triple at 230, Single at 260

Six weeks out: Triple at 220, Triple at 230, Double at 250

Seven weeks out: 3 doubles at 240

Eight weeks out: 3 triples at 225

This is an example that stresses starting well below your current 1 rep max and building up to exceed it once in the week before the meet.

Another significant difference between the peaking cycle and other cycles is that you will be doing very limited assistance work with the bulk of it being done in the early weeks. Toward the end of the cycle, close to the contest, you will cut back on assistance work, or eliminate it completely.

With that introduction, let me lay out the process of setting up your own peaking program.

Bench press

The first thing you will do is determine how long you want your peaking cycle to be. In the example, I'll use eight weeks. If you decide to use six weeks, you can simply eliminate the training recommended for the first two weeks.

For this example, I'll assume that the goal is a 315 bench press in a contest, with a current 1 rep max of 300.

Contest day: Planned attempts in the bench press: 280-305-315 (93%, 102%, 105%)

One week out: Single rep at 102% of current 1 rep max

Two weeks out: Single reps at 95% and 100% (of current 1 RM)

Three weeks out: Double at 85%   Single at 95%

Four weeks out: Double at 80%, Double at 85%

Five weeks out: Triple at 75%, Triple at 77%, Single at 80%

Six weeks out: Triple at 70%, Triple at 75%, Double at 83%

Seven weeks out: 3 doubles at 80%

Eight weeks out: 3 triples at 75%

Assistance Work

Following your bench press work, your assistance work will be primarily intended to ramp up your power, but not to burn you out.

On the eight-week cycle, I would recommend the following program:

Eight weeks out:
  Standing barbell press: 2 sets 5 reps
  Incline bench press: 2 sets 5 reps
  Power Cage lockouts: 4 lifts

Seven weeks out:
  Standing barbell press: 2 sets 5 reps
  Incline bench press: 2 sets 5 reps
  Power Cage lockouts: 4 lifts
  Barbell rowing: 2 sets 5 reps

Six weeks out:
  Standing barbell press: 2 sets 5 reps
  Incline bench press: 2 sets 5 reps
  Power cage lockouts: 4 lifts
  Barbell rowing: 2 sets 5 reps

Five weeks out:
  Standing dumbbell press: 2 sets 5 reps
  Barbell rowing: 2 sets 5 reps
  Power cage lockouts: 4 lifts

Four weeks out:
  Standing dumbbell press: 2 sets 5 reps
  Upright rowing: 2 sets 5 reps
  Power cage lockouts: 4 lifts

Four weeks out:
  Incline bench press: 2 sets 5 reps
  One arm rowing: 2 sets 5 reps
  Power cage lockouts: 4 lifts

Three weeks out:
  Incline bench press: 2 sets 5 reps
  One arm rowing: 2 sets 5 reps
  Power cage lockouts: 4 lifts

Two weeks out:
   Incline bench press: 1 set of 5 reps - light
   One arm rowing: 2 sets 5 reps - light
   Power cage lockouts: 2 lifts

One week out: (5-7 days before meet)
   Light bench press speed reps – (50% of 1 rep max) 4 sets of 2 reps
   Barbell rowing: 2 sets 5 reps – light

Your last workout before the meet should be 5-7 days before you lift. You must *minimize* the amount of training work you do. Remember, there is *nothing* you can do to get stronger in this last week, but a *lot* you can do to get weaker!

If you go to the gym, the best thing you can do is something relaxing or something that helps you recover. You need to put all your energy into the 9 attempts (3 on each lift) you will do at the contest, and most of what you do in the gym will detract from that.

During the final week before the contest, you should be checking your weight every day to make certain that you will be at the proper bodyweight on the day of the meet.

Some of you will have been cutting weight for a few weeks in preparation for the contest. I cover that in Chapter 16.

The biggest thing you can do to enhance your performance the week before the meet is *get lots of sleep.* Extra hours in bed asleep (not watching television) will give you a serious boost on the day of the meet.

The most important night to get extra rest is not the night before the contest, but the night TWO nights before you lift. For some reason the "night before the night before" has more of an impact on performance than the sleep immediately prior to the event.

If you sleep soundly and long for a week before the meet, you will be ready to do your best.

Now, go for that "PR".

Some Advanced Bench Press Training Techniques

The term "advanced" training approaches imply that there is some "secret" routine or technique that will magically produce all galaxy results where there had been only mediocre performance before.

Nothing could be further from the truth. In this case, advanced techniques are those that can help the *experienced* lifter who has mastered all the basic training methods. Advanced techniques are not a short cut to success.

As noted earlier, most of the advanced techniques require spotters. They cannot be undertaken without the help of other people. This is particularly true in the bench press where the potential for serious injury is more prominent than in the squat or the deadlift.

With that said, let me introduce some of the advanced techniques that can help the experienced lifter make progress.

Partial lifts using Boards and Blocks

There are multiple points in the bench press where a lifter can hit a sticking point. One of the ways to overcome these sticking points is to do partial bench presses. This is accomplished by placing boards or blocks of different thickness on the lifters chest while he or she is doing a bench press.

For example, say that the sticking point for a given lifter is about 2" (5 cm) above the chest. Placing a 2" board on the chest allows the lifter to lower a fully loaded bar to that point, and press upward. Thus it is possible to isolate the area where the lifter has difficulty.

This normally requires a training partner to hold the 2" board on the lifters chest while the exercise is being done. When heavy weights are being used, it is *mandatory* to have a spotter positioned at the midpoint in the lifting bar to rescue the lifter if he or she loses control of the bar.

Thicker blocks can be used to build strength in other parts of the bench press by using much heavier weights than could be pressed with a full range of motion. This helps to train strong lock outs and builds capacity in the stabilizer muscles to handle much heavier weights than could be done during the full bench press.

Again, someone must hold the boards on the lifters chest. With heavy overloads it is extremely important to have a spotter at the midpoint of the lifting bar to prevent serious injury if the lift cannot be completed.

The big advantage of using boards to lift the weight from different elevations off the chest is that unlike lifting in the power cage, the lifter must control both the descent of the weight and the press to lockout. Especially with heavy weights, controlling the weight is very demanding. This trains the stabilizer muscle groups in ways that are nearly impossible to duplicate in other ways.

Now a word on spotting and being safe. If you train heavy, you will need to have your spotters rescue you at least once during a workout...maybe more.

If you decide to use these techniques, it is *mandatory* that your training partners and spotters really know how to rescue you if you can't complete the lift.

The spotter right behind your head should keep his or her hands around the bar (but not touching) throughout this lift. In the bench press, when things go wrong, they go wrong so quickly it is impossible for anyone to move their hands fast enough to prevent a potentially horrendous injury.

If you are using really heavy weights, it is *mandatory* that you have a spotter on each end of the bar who will catch it if you lose control. It is also mandatory that the spotters are completely clear on what to do in the event the lifter loses control or yells for help.

The spotters on the ends of the bar should cup their hands with the fingers intertwined as shown in the photograph. They should always keep their hands immediately under the end of the bar while it is being lifted. As I said before, no one on earth can move their hands quickly enough to be of help if the bar suddenly goes out of control. If your hands are under the end of the bar, if a problem occurs the bar will simply drop into your ready hands.

If you lose control of the weight, the spotters on the end should "catch" the bar at whatever height it is when you lose control. They should not move it anywhere until you and the other spotters have explicitly talked about how to return the bar to the rack. If one of the end spotter pulls upward on the bar, while the other does not, the poor lifter on the bench is suddenly being crushed by an unstable and now unbalanced weight.

The spotter in the middle of the bar should be strong enough to deadlift the entire weight if you lose control. This is because if you lose control, they will have to catch the weight instantly. In other words, if you are doing partial bench presses with 500 pounds, the spotter in the middle should be able to deadlift that weight.

As you are astute, you will have noted that doing partial bench presses requires four spotters. One holding the boards, one in the middle of the bar, and two on the ends of the bar.

Doing partial lifts with boards is done with heavy weights, so you are never going to do more than two or three reps with this technique. I recommend that you do five sets or fewer using boards because you will tire quickly and the value of doing more work will be minimal or negative.

Using Elastic Bands

Using elastic bands in bench press training is primarily designed to work the stabilizer muscles that are critical for making a big lift. The bands create significant instability and force you to work hard to keep the bar in the "groove" for a proper bench press.

First of all, elastic bands come in different tension strengths. You should begin with a very light band to see how the pressure forces you to fight for control. When you become proficient with one band tension, you can move to the next level of tension.

There are two main exercises that I recommend you try using elastic bands. The first creates major instability in the lift off portion of the bench press.

In this movement, you attach the bands to the base of the bench and then loop them over the outside collar of the bar. This places maximum tension on the bar when it is on the rack and during the lift off. When you lower the bar to your chest, the tension on the bands diminishes, and you don't have to struggle for control.

In this first movement, I suggest you begin with only the bands and a bar without weights loaded on it. You will be amazed at how difficult it can be to lift the bar off the rack and then steady it for the descent even with no weight.

Because the band can create significant instability, it is imperative that you use a spotter when doing these movements. Although you are using relatively light weights, because of the instability, you can lose control of the bar and have a serious accident.

Add weight in small increments until you feel you can readily stabilize a weight that is 50% of your 1 rep maximum.

The second exercise creates instability throughout the entire bench press. This involves hanging two dumbbells or kettlebells off the area of the bar where you put the plates. Suspend dumbbells or kettlebells that are 25-35 pounds. This will be sufficient to create significant instability. The elastic band bounces the weight while you are holding or moving the bar. This will force you to mobilize all your stabilizer muscles to work against this constant instability.

You don't have to use much weight here as the principal objective is to activate the stabilizer muscles. You should start with only the dumbbell/kettlebell hanging from the bar, and gradually add weight as you become accustomed to controlling the bar. You should not aspire to do more weight than 40% of your 1 rep max.

It is most effective to use specific band exercises for a 4-week cycle. After that, your body has "learned" to mobilize the support muscles and you won't need to use these specific exercises for 6 months to a year.

Using Chains

Attaching chains to the bench press bar enables you to change the loaded weight throughout the lift. As you lower the bar, the chains pile up on the floor and essentially "de-load" the bar. It is lighter at the bottom than the top.

In my experience, this is a nice tool to have, but unless you belong to a gym where the owner has invested in these very expensive pieces of assistance equipment, the incremental value of using chains in training is minimal.

The amount of weight added to the bar will depend on the collection of chains available in your gym. Big chains weigh a lot and smaller ones weigh less. (Daaaah!) You should know how much each chain set adds to the bar weight. If no one knows how much each chain set weighs, go to the gym scale and weigh the link. (Note: be gentle with the scale when weighing chains or other heavy gym objects).

The chains need to be attached to the bar in such a way that they pile up on the floor as you lower the bar. Often you can hang them from a spring collar. If you simply drape them over the bar, they are nothing more than a barbell plate.

The basic way you use chains is to attach them to the ends of the lifting bar, and do 5 sets of 2-3 reps with perfect technique. Start with plates on the bar loaded to 70% or your 1 rep max. The chains will be extra weight. As you are stronger at the top of the lift, the chains will add weight to that part of the movement.

The chain will pile up on the floor as you lower the bar. When the bar is on your chest, pause and drive it up as rapidly as you can. As the chains come off the floor, the bar will get heavier and you will be working the lockout part of the lift.

As with bands, you should use chains in a 4-week cycle. Your body will adapt to them rapidly, and you need not use them more often than every six months to a year.

"Slingshot"

One of the more popular pieces of bench press training gear that has come along recently is an elastic strap that fits over each arm and goes across the chest. This provides a huge addition to the push off the chest.

These devices can be useful for the advanced lifter who wants to train with heavy weights and work on the lock out portion of the bench press.

This device is basically useless or outright detrimental to a novice or relatively inexperienced lifter. By providing lift off the chest from equipment, the device inhibits developing real strength in the lower part of the bench press.

However, for an experienced lifter the slingshot can help with lockout training.

Supportive Bench Press Shirts

The development of supportive shirts for the bench press has created massive increases in the amount of weight that people lift. In the era when everyone lifted in a t-shirt, bench presses were solid. However, as bench shirts became more and more high tech, the numbers lifted became mind boggling.

This book has been written with the assumption that most lifters will be training without support equipment such as high tech bench shirts. In powerlifting parlance, this is lifting "raw". In unequipped lifting, the objective is to make the body very strong rather than rely on equipment to create massively higher lifts.

However, because raw and equipped records and competitions are kept separate, many lifters have an interest in doing both raw and equipped lifting. For that reason, I'll discuss using bench shirts.

I'll start with the bottom line. That is, the technology of bench shirts is so complex and specialized that for anyone to get any benefit from this support gear it is absolutely necessary to work with a coach (or group of lifters) that really know how to get the most out of the gear.

In the "old days" (1980-90) most of us trained raw up until about a month before the contest and then put on the support gear. The incremental boost we got from the support gear was not so great that we had problems adapting to much higher weights.

Currently, if you lift competitively in support gear, it is usually advised that you train all the time using the support suits and shirts. That puts even more of a premium on training with a really knowledgeable coach.

Currently bench shirts cost between $150 and $300. Generally, the more expensive the shirt, the more effective it is.

There are some significant issues around wearing and using the shirt.

With the exception of "open back" shirts, it is impossible for a person to put on their own shirt. Adjusting the shirt for maximum effectiveness must be done by someone other than the person wearing the shirt. Very few coaches know how to adjust a shirt so that the wearer can get the most out of it. Thus, to make the shirt a worthwhile investment, it is absolutely necessary to find a coach or group of lifters who know how to put the shirt on, adjust it, and get the most out of it during a lift.

If you have worn a shirt before, and trained in it you know that it is *extremely* uncomfortable. When you use it to best effect, the shirt is downright painful.

Using shirts creates unusually dangerous situations when doing the bench press as the shirt, if properly adjusted, is always forcing your hands to move toward your face. This can result in you dropping the weight on your neck, so spotters are absolutely mandatory if you are lifting in a shirt.

Finally, it is impossible for a person wearing a shirt to get it off by themselves. In short, wearing a shirt and getting anything out of it requires at least one other person.

I should also mention that different lifting associations have different rules about which shirts are allowed in competition and which are not. The International Powerlifting Federation (IPF) allows single ply shirts only. Other associations allow double ply and even triple ply shirts.

If you intend to lift wearing support equipment, you must know what equipment is permitted in the association where you plan to compete.

Overall, I believe that your best focus for training is to lift without support gear *unless* you have the opportunity to train with a very knowledgeable group of lifters who use support equipment. Then you have the *choice* of training with our without support equipment.

For lifters over age 50, I would strongly recommend your primary training be "raw". It promotes great overall body strength and development, can be done on your own and is less dangerous.

I have lifted both raw and with support equipment because I had a group of top flight lifters and coaches available who knew how to best use the equipment. I enjoy raw training more because you don't have to worry about equipment related matters on every lift. Also, there are a full range of raw competitions available, so competing raw is easily accessible.

The bottom line on using advanced training techniques and equipment is that these can be useful if you are an experienced lifter. I would recommend that you spend at least two years training and competing raw before considering using support equipment.

Chapter 9

Deadlift: Pulling Monster Iron – Technique and Basic Assistance Exercises

The deadlift comes last in a competition and it is the lift that generally determines who posts the best total. It is possible to put up some really big numbers here, and overcome some problems with the squat and bench press. In short, it is a *really* important lift.

Since the deadlift appears mechanically simple, some lifters seem to believe that simply "pulling like hell" will yield a maximum lift. No way....

Like the other powerlifts, deadlifting looks easy to do. In terms of lifting technique, it is looks like all you do is bend over and stand up with the weight in your hands. This is true only if you don't care how much you lift. Maximizing your performance involves mastering a lot of small but very critical lifting techniques.

Mastering the *small details* of performance is the difference between being a mediocre lifter and reaching your full potential.

Over my 25 years of competing and being a referee, I have seen a lot of lifters give away many pounds of performance with lousy technique. When I was officiating I saw almost every lifter do all their lifts in a meet. It always amazed me the performance gulf between those lifters who had good technique and those that simply "pulled like hell".

When you consider the time you invest in training, consider this: it takes the same amount of training time to be mediocre or to be really good. You can use your training time to develop great technique, or to *perfect your mistakes*.

In the section that follows, I'm going to go through the lift in great detail. I would strongly suggest that you not breeze over any of the details. Each of them can be worth a few pounds on your lift. Put several of them together and you have a much bigger lift than you may have thought possible.

Conventional or Sumo Style?

Conventional style deadlifting means that the feet are placed shoulder width or narrower. In the sumo style deadlift, the feet are placed wider than the shoulders. How wide the feet are spaced depends on how tall the lifter is, and the point where they feel they can generate the most leverage. Both conventional and sumo style lifters use the same shoulder width grip.

I have never found any convincing evidence that one style was better than the other. The choice of one style over another seems to boil down to individual body mechanics and leverages. In other words, your physical frame.

Persons such as myself who are relatively tall with long arms seem to do best with the conventional style deadlift. People who have short trunks and relatively shorter arms seem to do best with the sumo style.

You will have to make your own decision about which you want to use. If you are relatively new to powerlifting, I strongly suggest you start out using the conventional style deadlift technique. When you have a few years of experience, you may want to experiment with the sumo style.

The reason I suggest this is that the sumo style lift is harder to keep "in the groove" during a pull. Because the lifters base is spread out, there is more chance for unwanted twisting to undercut a solid pull.

If you are an experienced powerlifter, then you have probably practiced one style more than the other. If you want to experiment, try the "other" style for a month long training cycle to see if it appears to offer any advantages to you.

Personally, I used the conventional style my entire lifting career. I did experiment with the sumo on several occasions, but found that I could not lift nearly as much as with conventional style. I attribute this to my individual body mechanics.

Equipment

As noted earlier, powerlifters who use support gear (equipped) and those who lift without support equipment (raw) do not compete against each other. Support gear offers significant advantages in the squat and the bench press. Squat suits and bench shirts have added some staggering amounts to each of these lifts.

For example, some (very large) men can bench press 800-900 pounds using very thick special bench shirts. The same lifters will usually struggle to bench 550-600 pounds when lifting raw.

Unlike the bench press and the squat, deadlift suits have not produced a dramatic difference between "raw" (no support gear) and equipped lifts. The amount most people are able to deadlift raw is not much different than when using support gear.

Like the support gear used in squatting and bench pressing, the suits and shirts evolve over time. Generally, the support gear becomes more and more specialized and can only be used to good advantage with the assistance of a coach who is completely knowledgeable in the most recent changes in the equipment.

The reason for this is that the suits (and shirts) are extremely tight and *very* uncomfortable. It often takes two people to help force a lifter into their squat suit or bench press shirt. Because the support suits and shirts are so tight, they must be adjusted for a *perfect* fit which will force the lifter to move the bar in one "groove".

In many cases the support equipment is so difficult to get on and to fit properly, that without a coach or training partners who are completely up to date (as in the last 90 days) using the gear may put the trainee at great risk, or severely limit their what they can lift.

In the deadlift, there are new deadlift suits that require a nearly complete change in the way lift is performed in order to get anything from the support gear. The results of using deadlift suits are mixed at best, with a few lifters able to get some advantage from the gear.

On the other hand, using deadlift suits has also created circumstances where the lift must be done perfectly, or it fails completely. This changes deadlifting from a relatively predictable lift to a "high risk" adventure.

Unless you train with a group of lifters who are very sophisticated about the use of support gear, you should be training for "raw" lifting. I have nothing against using support gear, but from my experience lifting both raw and in support gear, I can assure you that unless you have a really experienced coach who knows how to use the latest "stuff", you are putting yourself in harm's way if you try to use support gear.

Because the suits and so specialized and hard to use, while offering little advantage, all the advice I offer will be on raw lifting. For you to be able to pull "big iron" it is essential that you train your *unsupported body* (aka. "raw"). Regardless of whether you use support gear, training "raw" is the key to having a big deadlift.

Critical Equipment for Deadlift Training

A good lift, in a meet or in training, begins *before* you get up to the bar. You have to have the right equipment or you are throwing away a huge amount of weight that you might be able to lift.

Even though you are lifting raw, it is critical that you have certain essential things for you to excel at the deadlift. These may sound like simple items, but they will have a profound impact on how well you are able to lift.

The absolutely essential equipment you need to have:

- Chalk for your hands
- Proper lifting belt
- Proper footwear
- Shin protection

There is one product that will always help you on your biggest lifts….CHALK. That is right. Believe it or not, this humble substance will add 150-200 pounds to your grip. If you can't hang on to the bar, you can't lift the weight. You should always use chalk on your heavy pulls in training and obviously in a contest. Before you attempt a deadlift in practice or a meet, put chalk on your hands.

The product you should have is called "gymnastics chalk". It is available in some large sporting goods stores, and on the internet. You should always have some in your workout bag, preferably in a sealed food storage container so that it doesn't get on your other gear.

If you don't already know, many gyms will prohibit the use of chalk. This is because too many inconsiderate people before you made a mess with chalk and didn't clean it up. If your gym bans chalk, use it very discreetly and clean up any dust you may leave.

If your gym does not ban chalk, use it carefully and clean up after yourself. The gym owner will be glad to see you, and it will set an example for others.

When you are pulling iron that is near your max, a powerlifting belt will help support your core. But, you should not rely on the belt for support until you are within 90% of your one rep maximum lift. Using the belt with lighter weights will *make you weaker.*

By training without support gear you "build in" support strength in all parts of your bod to help you pull your max deadlift. Using support gear when training with lighter weights means you will become dependent on the gear and not develop all the support strength you need.

Far too many novice lifters strap on a lifting belt as soon as they finish warm ups. This is a self-defeating practice, because it makes you *weaker.* The essence of your training is to make your body strong and not rely on artificial support devices.

Powerlifting belts are highly specialized pieces of equipment that are available only on the internet from powerlifting suppliers. They are made of double ply leather only and are roughly 4" (10 cm) wide and 3/8" (10-13mm) thick. They will have either a "lever" style belt, or a conventional style buckle. They are *never* sold in stores, or at least I have never seen any in the 25 years I competed. For a list of suppliers, see my website at www.MidLifeHardBody.com.

There are many "imposter" belts out there.

The thin brown lifting belts sold in sporting goods stores are for Olympic style lifting. The Olympic style belts are single ply lightweight leather and no more than 4" wide in the back. They are narrow in the front, and do not give you the type of abdominal support you need for powerlifting.

There are also some belts that are very wide in the back. They are largely useless for any type of lifting. These have been around since the 50's and for unknown reasons still survive as a product. Like a lot of "sporting goods" equipment, this belt may have been designed by people who don't lift anything heavier than a sandwich.

More junk: Recently there are a number of nylon belts, or belts with Velcro type fasteners. None of these are legal for competition and most are simply cheesy crap for the Ken and Barbie crowd. Don't waste your money.

My strong personal preference in powerlifting belts are the ones with a lever buckle. They can be preset to a given waist size and all you need to do to tighten them is push on the lever. Trying to struggle with a conventional buckle when you are getting ready for a big lift is a huge waste of energy and can be a significant distraction.

Now….perhaps the single most important item in your deadlifting wardrobe….footwear.

One of the biggest things you need to know is that your <u>footwear</u> has a massive impact on how much you can deadlift. You should always lift wearing shoes that have **<u>flat soles</u>**. A shoe that has any sort of raised heel will throw you forward out of your most powerful lifting groove. You should *never* lift in athletic shoes with a raised heel. This includes Olympic lifting shoes.

Another thing you don't want in your shoes is any padding added for shock absorption. You want a shoe with a sole as thin as you can find. The padding creates problems for you because it means you will be pulling off an unstable surface. The last thing you want to do is be fighting for your balance when pulling a heavy weight.

The padding also creates a problem because it means you have to lift this heavy weight *an extra inch or more* than if you were lifting with bare feet. If you are wearing athletic shoes with an inch of sole between you and the platform, it means that in the most difficult part of the lift, the initial pull off the ground, you have to move the bar from an inch *below* where you would start if you were barefoot.

For conventional style lifters, far and away the best "shoes" to use when deadlifting are ballet slippers…often sold as deadlift slippers. They have the advantage of being flat, and having only a thin strip of rubber between your foot and the floor. These slippers are the choice of big time lifters all over the world. They are legal for use in competition, and perfect for training.

Sumo style lifters often opt for wrestling shoes since with a wide stance, slippers may tend to roll over. Tightly laced wrestling shoes will stay stable with wide foot spacing.

Finally, there is the issue of protecting your shins. You will want to wear soccer sox or long training pants to protect your shins from being scraped by the bar. If you do the lift properly, the bar will brush against your shins until you have pulled it to your knees. Being scraped up is both unsightly and painful. You will have to wear sox that come up just below the knee during competition, so training with them makes sense.

You may want to wear thin soccer shin guards during training. I did this for years since lots of deadlift workouts can leave you with painfully scraped shins. There is nothing cool about the look, and scraped shins tend to hurt even when you are not rubbing something against them.

While there is really no support equipment that will help you add much to your deadlift, there are some items sold that will *drastically diminish* what you can pull.

Lifting "straps" supposedly help you grip a heavier weight than you could otherwise pull. I would strongly suggest you NEVER use these. Straps will destroy any chance you have to develop a powerful grip. Your good buddy chalk is the only thing you should use when lifting a heavy bar.

Lifting "gloves" have little use other than keeping your hands warm if you lift in an unheated garage during northern winters. Gloves are one of those workout gadgets dreamed up by the Vice President in Charge of Useless Products in a sporting goods firm to sell to the unwary. Like straps, gloves will subvert your grip strength. You don't want to look like the Incredible Hulk, but have the grip of Mother Teresa. Besides….you can't wear gloves in a contest.

There are some "shoes" sold as "powerlifting shoes" that are essentially a $120 version of the same thing you could buy for $10 (maybe $20) at Goodwill Industries. These shoes are basically old time basketball shoes (minus the style cache') and the only thing that makes them useful for powerlifting is that they don't have a raised heel. Feet flat on the floor…and no padding between you and the deck.

Some lifters want to put baby powder on their thighs before a heavy lift to help the bar slide up their legs. Personally, I have never found that this helps much, but it does make a mess. It is almost guaranteed to make you very unpopular with gym owners who don't care for people who make a mess for them to clean up. If the gym owner thinks you are a "powder pig", this is not an indicator that you will be training there over the long term.

Now that you have chalk, a powerlifting belt, tall sox and proper footwear, you are ready to walk on the platform either in training or competition.

I will remind you that the things you do in training will be the things you do in a competitive meet. So, it is to your benefit to do your training lifts exactly the same way as you would in a contest. This begins with your preparation to go on the platform.

Begin by putting chalk on your hands. Find the amount that is optimal for you. Some lifters use more than others. You need to find the amount that gives you the best grip.

IF you are using a lifting belt, tighten it *before* you walk onto the platform to lift.

As I have noted elsewhere, I strongly recommend that you NOT use a lifting belt until you are lifting a weight that is 90% of your one rep maximum. You want to build the strength of your core muscles to support a heavy lift. Using a belt on light lifts weakens you.

When you have chalk on your hands, your belt in place and your mind focused on pulling the weight, it is time to walk on the platform.

Deadlifting Technique: Step by Step

Getting tight to pull big iron

Developing maximum tension in your body before you pull a deadlift is a skill you need to practice the same way you would practice shooting in basketball. It is critical to your success, so deliberate practice is mandatory.

You should practice building tension in your body every deadlift workout. Like developing other sport skills, you will get better and better if you practice this regularly.

Now, the caveat. Most lifters will not bother to practice getting tight for the deadlift if they don't see instant results. Practicing getting tight may also look a little strange to your training partners. For these reasons, a lot of people will ignore getting tight and train as they always have. Don't be that person!

Like the squat and the bench press, every time you do a deadlift, regardless of the weight, use *perfect* technique. Treat you 135 lb warm up the same way you would treat your 635 attempt.

Walk up to the bar, and set your feet in position so that the bar is touching your shins.

Conventional style foot position will be shoulder width or narrower. The object is to pull off what feels like a single point on the floor. Your feet will be 12"-15" inches apart. All your weight will be on the *inside half* of your foot.

Sumo style foot position will be either the same you use to squat, or very wide so that your feet are within a foot of the plates on the lifting bar. Your weight will be on the inside half of your foot.

When you have your feet in place, your next move is to get tight. You do this while standing erect over the bar.

Here is a way to practice getting tight for deadlifting.

Begin by standing erect with your shins against the lifting bar. Begin by taking a deep breath, driving air into your abdomen. Hold the breath throughout the entire lift.

Dig your toes into the floor. Feel as if you are rooted into the floor. Tighten your calf muscles, then pull your quads upward. Pinch your glutes together. Tighten your abs and lock down against the air in your belly. Tighten your back.

Flex your shoulders and pull them back. Flex your upper arms, and pull the muscles in your forearms up toward your elbows. Tighten your neck and shoulders and clench your teeth. Keep your back flat. At this point your body should be completely tense.

Now….you begin to descend to grasp the bar…..This is where you start dealing with unfamiliar feelings.

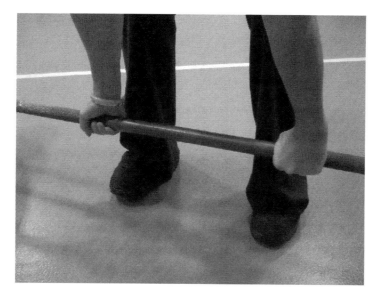

Deadlift grip

You have to stay tight as you descend. This takes practice.

When you go down to the bar, you should literally feel like a big hand is pushing you down. You should "pull" yourself down building more and more tension in your muscles as you go lower and lower.

You descend by pushing your rear end back as if you were going to sit in a chair. As you descend, you should feel the pressure in your abdomen build as you compress the air in your abdomen. The compressed air in your abdomen will contribute to the force that helps you pull the loaded bar off the floor.

Look down at your hands by lowering your eyes, and not by bending your head forward. Keep your head erect as much as possible, and keep the back flat.

Get your grip on the bar, and adjust your hip height to the angle that is optimal for you. You should try to crush the bar with your grip.

At this point, you should be in perfect position for the pull with your body completely tense.

The deep set up

Your entire body is under maximum tension. Remember, *any muscle that is relaxed during the pull is like a leak in a hydraulic system.* You cannot afford any "leaks".

The image you should have in mind is that your body is a giant spring compressed under tension.

Your hips should be at the optimal elevation for you to get the strongest pull. This will vary from one individual to another, and you will have to find your own optimal hip angle. Your back must be flat. Pull your shoulders *back*. Keep your head erect, staring straight ahead.

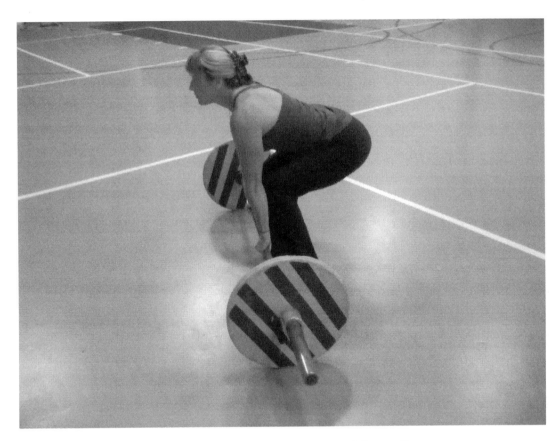

Proper position for the start of the pull

You are still holding your breath. The air in your belly will compress, creating pressure that will help you lift the bar.

Again, you doing your best to create maximum tension as you go down to the start position. This eccentric "loading" of your muscles means that when you begin coming up, it will have the effect of a big spring uncoiling as you move the bar upward.

You should have a narrow grip on the bar. Right where the knurling begins is a good place to aim for. The wider the grip, the greater the distance off the floor you must lift the bar.

Your grip will be one hand with the palm facing back toward you, and the other palm facing forward. This grip will allow you to lift vastly more weight than if both palms face the same way. When you have your hands in the right place, squeeze the bar hard. Remember, you are recruiting every muscle you can.

Your shins should be touching the bar. Your shins should be perpendicular to the floor (straight up and down). When you are properly set for the pull, the bar will be directly below your chin.

It is critical that your shoulders are pushed back, and positioned so they are behind the bar on the floor.

Your back should be absolutely flat, with no bend or bow anywhere. This is the most powerful position your back can be in for a big lift. You MUST keep your back flat throughout the lift.

Your shoulders must be rolled back. Your hips should be relatively low so that the first pull on the bar is done with your legs and abdominal muscles.

Your entire body is under maximum tension ready to uncoil upward. Now comes the pull.

The Pull

If you have set up properly, your body should feel like it is ready to explode from the pressure generated by the breath compressed in your lungs, and the tension you have loaded on your muscles getting down to grip the bar.

Now you begin a series of steps that you *must* do if you are going to get a maximum lift.

Before you actually move the bar off the floor, pull upward with about 100 pounds of force. You want to make the bar bend a little *before* the weight comes off the ground. Putting upward pressure on the bar is *huge!* Doing this means you will not have to move the entire weight from a dead stop. It will make every weight you pull seem much lighter.

As you this tension on the bar, feel like you are driving your feet into the floor. The sensation should feel is that you are "pushing" the weight upward by extending your legs.

The pressure on your feet should be on the inside half of your foot. That is where power is generated. The outside half is for balance.

There is a "groove" right next to your body where you can generate the maximum pulling force. That is where you want to keep the bar throughout the pull. To keep the bar "in the groove" you keep it against your body during the entire pull.

You should *never* allow the bar to drift forward, nor should you allow your shoulders to go forward over the bar. Your shoulders must always be *back* of the bar.

You begin the pull with 100 pounds of tension on the bar. Pushing your feet into the floor, *slowly* move the bar off the floor. You should think of your body being in low gear...putting out *max power*!!

You should *never* jerk the bar off the floor. In order to jerk the bar up, your body has to be relaxed, so you won't have the advantage of the loaded tension in your muscles. Jerking will also mean that you get a big surge of power followed by almost immediate collapse. You will only move the bar about a half inch before you completely lose power.

As you pull the bar up your shins you should keep your hips low, back flat, and head erect. It is critical that you keep driving your shoulders *back*. If you don't keep your shoulders back, the bar may drift forward out of the groove and you are screwed!

Your head should always be erect. You should focus your gaze on a point in the back of the room and keep it there throughout the pull. This will help keep your head in proper position. You should *never* look down as it will tend to cause your back to bend forward. If you exaggerate head position by looking up, it will also distort your pull and possibly cause balance problems.

You *must* keep the bar tight against your legs. If the bar drifts away from your body, you lose leverage rapidly and your pull becomes very weak.

Once the weight has moved a few inches off the floor, you should think about pulling the weight as fast as you can. It will not be very fast, but this is a technique for putting 100% effort into the pull.

You should NOT feel the lift in your lower back. If you do, your butt is up too high and you are not getting a good push with the legs.

The pull must be smooth and the bar can never descend, even a little bit, at any point in the lift. You cannot "hitch" or stop and jerk the bar upward.

When the bar clears your knees, pull it back into your thighs and begin to push your hips forward. Keep the bar against your body. If it drifts forward, you will lose a dramatic amount of leverage.

You cannot re-bend the knees at any point. This "dipping" under the bar is cause for "no lift". Once you have straightened the knees, they must stay straight.

Keep your shoulders back throughout the pull, keeping your back flat. Never allow your back to round over at any point in the lift.

Stand erect and straighten your knees. You will have to stand completely erect in competition with no bend in the knees. Do this in every practice and you won't have to think about it in a contest.

When you are fully erect, you can release your breath. Now, lower the weight to the floor under complete control. You literally <u>set the weight back on the floor.</u> NEVER drop the weight. In a contest this is cause for disqualification. You MUST always lower the weight under complete control and set it down.

The practice of "dumping" weights has become popular since Cross Fit and some other gyms have introduced Olympic style lifting using rubber "bumper" plates. This allows people to drop weights when the lift is complete without the risk of broken metal plates.

Recently we have seen an epidemic of dropping weights from various altitudes in gyms across the country. Rubber plates have made it possible for even Bart Simpson to toss a barbell on the floor with the utter distain normally reserved for a Russian Heavyweight Olympic champion.

While this display of "attitude" might be considered a form of expressing your inner self in the Ever so Perfect Millennials Gym, dropping a weight in powrlifting is both seriously lame…..and *against the rules.*

Dropping weights in powerlifting only happens when you lose your grip or have an accident. Dumping any powerlift is quite dangerous and is something you should never do. You are NOT doing Olympic lifting. It is a completely different sport. Even if you do powerlifting training in a Cross Fit gym (as I have) you NEVER dump your weights.

In powerlifting *real* men and women lower their weights under control. If you are going to try to lift big iron, act like the adults not like the pimple squeezers. So…. hang on to the iron…all the way to the floor.

You will need to practice all aspects of proper deadlifting technique and use it on every pull you do. It will make a big difference on how much you can pull in any one lift, and will allow you to keep making progress. If you have poor technique, this creates an artificially low ceiling on how high you can go. So…practice good technique on every rep.

A few (high risk) technique oddities

The technique I have described above is guaranteed to help you build great power and reach your full potential. It is used by 99% of the top flight lifters. But, just so you don't think I have overlooked something, I want to let you know about some unusual techniques that I have seen that on the surface may appear to have some merit.

One of them is lifting with a rounded upper back. I have seen one or two top flight lifters use this, but I should warn you it is used only by a few lifters who developed this style over decades. It has no particular advantage, and is probably dangerous to most lifters. Stay away from the rounded back.

Another unusual technique I have seen (only one top flight lifter I know uses this), is to run up to the bar, grab it and pull. This supposedly generates a lot of explosiveness. However, like the "grip and rip" technique I discussed earlier, the normal effect is to generate great force for a second or two, the go to complete collapse.

As I said, I have seen one top flight lifter use this technique. Because he practiced it all the time, and had done it for 20+ years, it worked for him. However, because of the speed that he used running up to the bar, there was always the chance for something unusual to go wrong.

In one instance, I saw this lifer grab a deadlift and pull like mad...only to find that one of his fingers had gotten stuck inside a shoe lace loop. Naturally, the lift came crashing back to earth very quickly. This happened in an international championship meet and cost him a big lift.

Master the proper technique and you will be able to lift monster weights. Don't search for gimmicks or short cuts.

Just so you know that I practice what I preach, here is a photo of me pulling a 400+ lift during training.

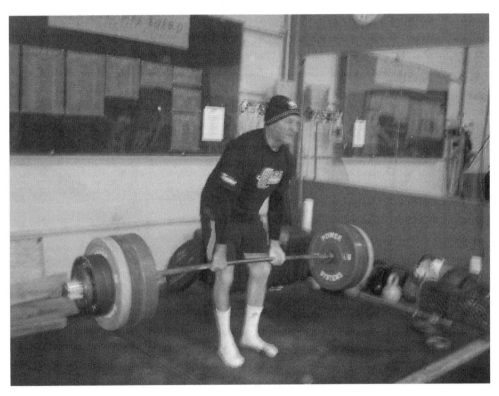

Core Deadlift Assistance Exercises

I have grouped the main deadlift assistance exercises in one section, because you will be using them in more than one cycle.

You will be doing one or two of the core assistance exercises in every deadlift training cycle.
In addition, you will do one or more additional assistance exercises that I'll describe in the section on each cycle.

It is also worth noting that deadlift training is very synergistic with squat training in that both place major demands on the legs, back, core and stabilizer muscles. Doing one heavy squat session and one heavy deadlift session each week works a lot of the same muscles.

Assistance work for the deadlift is designed to train parts of the lift that are unique to the pull.

As a general rule, I recommend that you do heavy assistance work during periods when you are some months away from a contest. When you are doing heavy deadlift training (peaking for a contest or a max attempt), you should back off on the assistance work.

Remember, you will get stronger by lifting heavy weights *and recovering!*

In my opinion, there are five deadlift assistance exercises that can have a major impact on building a big pull. I advise including one or two of them in each training cycle, depending on what portion of the lift is the weakest for you. All of them should be done at some time during the year.

- Rumanian Deadlift
- Deadlift off a raised surface
- Good morning exercise
- Power Cage deadlifts (partial lifts)

These are the assistance movements that I believe will contribute the *most* to building power.

You will do one or two of these high payoff exercises in any given training cycle. Over the course of a year, and multiple training cycles, you will wind up doing all of them.

Both squatting and deadlifting take a huge amount of energy and place big demands on the central nervous system. It is really critical that you not over train on "assistance" work.

In my experience, most lifters have a tendency is to do too much heavy work, and not allow for adequate recovery. This is to prevent "crashing" from over work

Your body does not distinguish between regular deadlift workouts and "assistance" work. You will need to be aware that too much hard work can result in slowing your gains, plateaus, and sometimes going into reverse.

With that in mind, here are the exercises that I believe will give you the most benefit.

Deadlift off a Block

One of the movements that helps you get the weight started off the floor is to deadlift with your feet on a low block. This creates the effect of starting to pull the bar below normal bar height.

The block need only be 2" or 3" in height. Anything higher distorts your form so much that the training benefit is reduced.

As you can see in the photograph, you can use a 45 lb barbell plate for your "elevation". You don't want to pull from too great a height, because it distorts your lifting form. Besides, you get most of the benefit from lifting off an elevated platform from the first inch or two.

Going below the normal starting position will help develop power for the start of the lift when you are fighting to overcome the forces of gravity and inertia. The rule in physics that says "a body at rest tends to remain at rest" is will never be clearer to you than when you begin to pull on a deadlift bar.

Deadlifting from a little below the normal starting point can help you be better prepared to overcome the forces of gravity.

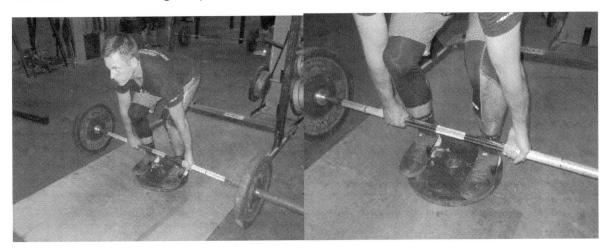

Deadlift standing on a barbell plate

Rumanian Deadlift

If the good morning exercise looked like a bad squat, the Rumanian Deadlift looks like a poorly done straight leg deadlift. In reality, this is one of the greatest builders of lower back strength ever devised.

Load the bar as if you were going to do a regular deadlift. When you stand over the bar, your shins will be against the bar and your feet in position for a conventional deadlift.

Bend over and grip the bar, keeping your back flat, with your knees slightly bent, and your tail end elevated...or "way up in the air".

Pull the bar off the floor and stand erect. Your knees should be flexed during the pull, *not straight*. It is really important that your back be flat during the pull.

This will really tax your lower back. That is the purpose of the lift.

You will want to do 3 sets of 3 reps with a reasonably demanding weight. You will build super back strength, and go a long way toward protecting yourself against injury.

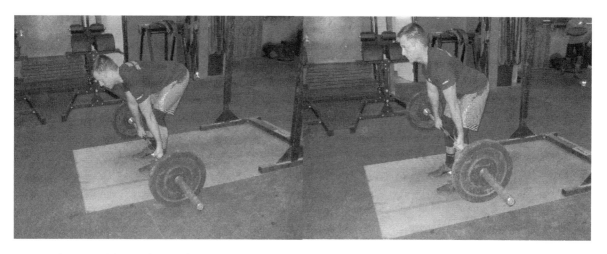

Starting position – hips elevated   **Mid-pull – standing up with slight bend in knee**

Good Morning Exercise

This is one of those movements that is practiced infrequently, in large measure because it is hard to do. It also looks somewhat strange. To the uninitiated it can look like a really bad squat.

This is one of those movements that is practiced infrequently, in large measure because it is hard to do. It also looks somewhat strange. To the uninitiated it can look like a really bad squat.

However, this movement will give you great strength, and you should do them regularly throughout the year as part of our deadlift assistance training.

Begin by putting a bar on your back as if you were going to do a competition squat. Position the bar in the same place you would for a squat, and *never* up on your neck.

Keeping your back flat, bend forward at the waist until your chest is nearly parallel to the floor. You should bend your knees slightly to keep your balance, and keep your head up.

You should feel a strong pull in your glutes and hamstrings. That is where most of the work should be done.

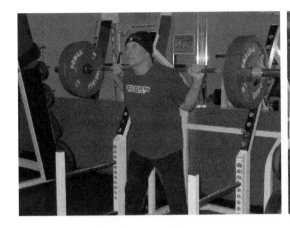 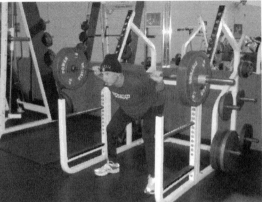

Starting position   **Bend forward at the waist**

You can probably see what I mean when I say it looks like a really lame squat. However, all the tension and work is being done by the core, and the posterior power chain.

As I said, this exercise is not practiced very often, so there is a good chance you have not done it. Learn to do it well and you will get a really strong core and backside. While you are learning it, start out with a weight you can manage with relative ease for 3 sets of 3 reps.

Your goal is to do 5 sets of 3 reps with a weight that is slightly difficult to handle. You will gradually increase the weight as you become more skilled at the movement and as you get stronger.

However, this movement will give you great strength, and you should do them regularly throughout the year as part of our deadlift assistance training.

Power Cage Training

The power cage is one of the great tools that allow you to *safely* handle huge weights. In the squat section of this book you saw how the power cage allowed you to do super heavy partial movements and isometric movements. In this section I'll talk about these types of movements for deadlift training.

Partial Deadlifts

A "partial" deadlift is one where you do one part of the lift, not the entire deadlift movement. With partial lifts you handle much heavier weights than you could with a regular deadlift. These big overloads help build total body power, pulling strength, and make your regular full deadlifts seem light by comparison.

Doing partials involves positioning the support pins so that you begin lifting bar at different heights. You lift the bar starting from different heights and complete the lift to full lock out.

There are two basic positions for doing partial deadlifts: below the knees and above the knees.

Safety Issues

Before doing heavy partial lifts in a cage, there are some safety issues you need to know.

You will be using *very heavy* weights and it is important that you keep them under control. The power cage is a very sturdy device, designed to keep you safe while moving big iron. However, if you abuse the equipment, it will break.

Remember, the faster a bar heavily loaded bar is moving, the more force it generates. (Remember: force = mass x acceleration). The more you keep the bar under control, the less likely that you will create any forces that will break the support rods or any part of the power cage.

For all your partial lifts be sure to do the following:

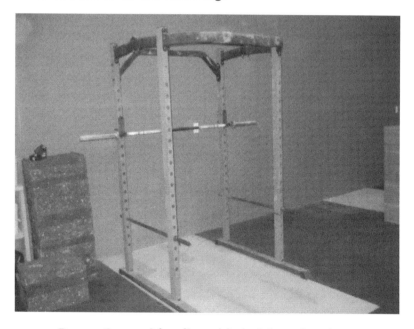

Power Cage with adjustable height safety bars

You will be placing the deadlift bar on support rods that go through holes of the front and back upright ribs of the power cage. There is a support rod on each side of the cage. The holes in the uprights are drilled at standard intervals so that the lifting bar can be supported parallel to the floor at different heights.

In the picture below you can see a typical power cage. The bar is resting on brackets set at a height where a user could take it for doing squats. The support rods are inserted at a level where a squatter could leave the bar if they could not come up from the low point in a squat.

You can position the support rods at different heights. In squatting the rods were positioned at a place that would catch the bar if you could not come up with the squat. You can also use the rods as starting points for different exercises.

In deadlift training you are going to use the support rods to position the lifting bar at heights where you want to begin the lift. A couple of basic rules apply for positioning the loaded bar on the rods.

First, position the bar you are going to lift as close to the front (or back) upright of the cage as you can. This will mean that the heavily loaded bar will be resting on the support rod within an inch or a few cm of where the rod goes into the hole in the upright support. The purpose of this is to position the lifting bar at the location where it has the greatest support.

You should *never* position the bar in the middle of the support rod. This is the weakest section of the rod. Since you will be using big weights, there is a chance you may bend (or break) the support pin. This is very dangerous.

 The second safety rule is that when you have locked out the pull, lower the bar back to the support rod under control. There are two reasons for this. The first is that if you suddenly relax at the completion of your lock out, you may be seriously injured by a big weight going into free fall. The second is that it can be really unsafe for you and others around the cage to drop a heavily loaded bar.

Dropping a heavily loaded bar onto the metal support rods will create a dramatic sounding crash…but is *very* dangerous. If you drop a heavy bar, even from a few inches, it can snap or bend the support rod. If it breaks one or both of the rods, you have no control over the weight and it may throw you like a rag doll in any direction, or land on you. You may also have to contend with chunks of flying metal. In short…a very bad scene.

Deadlifting from just below the knees

One of the hardest parts of the deadlift is getting the bar past the knees. A major "sticking point" occurs just below the knee when the pulling leverages change slightly. Doing partial deadlifts from the point just below the knees can really build strength to drive past the sticking point.

Set the support rod at a level so that the barbell you are pulling is an inch (3 cm) below the bottom of the kneecap. By starting the bar at this position, you can directly work on one of the most difficult parts of the pull.

Your goal will be to pull as heavy a weight as possible starting from this position and going to a full lock out. Do this movement for a single rep, or at most two reps. You will only do this for two or at most three sets.

Because each of us has slightly different leverages, each lifter will have to experiment to find their beginning poundage. A good place to start is at about 80% of your 1 rep maximum full deadlift. Add weight until you have to put out about 95% effort to do a single rep.

Doing more than three sets (singles or doubles) will really tax your central nervous system, and you will really drastically diminish the value of this work by doing too much.

Set up for the pull with the same technique you would use when pulling a regular deadlift. You will get the most benefit if your technique on the partial lift is identical to what it would be in a full deadlift.

Before you start, make certain your body is under full tension the way it would be if you were doing a full deadlift. You can use your lifting belt, or not. If you have been pulling heavy for several years, forget the belt. If you are in the first few years of doing heavy training, use the belt.

Heavy pulls are the greatest builder of grip strength ever devised. Put chalk on your hands. As I said earlier, chalk will add 150-200 pounds to what you can hang on to. *Never ever* use lifting straps or lifting gloves. These will destroy any chance you have to build a powerful grip.

Set your feet, take your normal grip, completely tighten your body, crush the bar with your hands, put your shoulders back and then apply about 100 pounds of upward force on the bar. You are now ready to do the lift. Pull the bar to full lockout position and hold it for about two seconds, then lower it under control to the support pins.

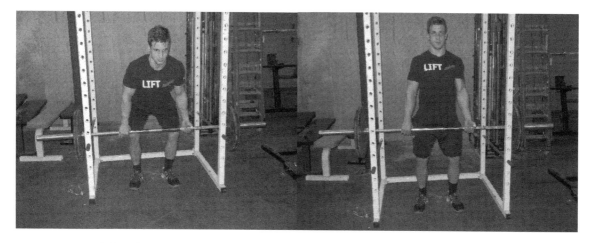

Partial deadlifts in the power rack: starting and finishing positions

If you do two reps, set the bar down on the support pins after the first rep and begin the pull from a dead stop. *Do not ever* bounce the bar off the support pins using the "touch and go" style move. This is basically useless for your training purposes.

Lockouts

This is one of the most important of the cage exercises, because you will be able to use a huge overload from your normal deadlift. For example, if your best deadlift is 400 pounds, you may eventually work up do doing lock outs with 600 pounds (or more).

This exercise will make your regular deadlift seem light. It will also give you the grip strength you need to be a top flight deadlifter.

In this exercise, you will set the bottom pins so that the barbell is just *above* your knees. This is the "finishing" part of the lift.

Do your set up with the bar against your legs, shoulders back, completely tighten your body, crush the bar with your hands, apply 100 pounds of upward force, and pull up. Stand erect with the bar in your hands to the full lockout position.

Hold the lift for 2 seconds, and lower it back to the starting point under full control.

Again, do singles with this lift because it is using a huge amount of weight, and puts a lot of strain on your whole body and central nervous system.

I strongly suggest you keep the number of sets to three as you will burn out quickly.

The lock out can add a lot to your full deadlift, but not if you over train. Allow for good recovery and you will get a lot from this exercise.

A Creative Use of the Power Rack

The legendary Paul Anderson used the power rack to great advantage during his almost mythical reign as the world strongest man. One of the techniques he often suggested (from his own training) was to use the power rack to gradually adapt to heavy poundage in the squat and deadlift.

Anderson's technique can be adapted to your training. In the conventional style deadlift, begin by taking a weight that is 5-10% heavier than you can do a regular off the floor lift. Place the barbell on the power rack pins at a height where you can lock the weight out with about 85% effort on two reps.

Over several weeks, you will gradually start the lift at a lower and lower position by changing the height where you start the pull. You are in essence training yourself to work into a full deadlift by moving the same weight lower and lower in the power cage.

Because you cannot lift the big weight initially, you want to make small changes so your body can adapt. It is desirable that you change where you start the pull by roughly a half inch each time you lower the weight.

Since most power racks have holes 2" apart or more, the best technique I have found is to cut pieces of half inch plywood so that you can stand on them when you lift. This is the same as lowering the pin in half inch increments. To get changes of more than a half inch, simply stack the pieces of plywood on top of each other until you are ready to move the support pin 2".

You have not developed the strength to lift a big weight from 2" lower than you could do initially. You can continue to work your way down the starting point in the power rack using the plywood platform to make small changes in your starting point.

This technique would be hard to use with the sumo style deadlift unless you cut the plywood pieces long enough so that you have one piece on which you place both feet. If the plywood is in two pieces, it will probably slide apart when you try to lift.

Remember, the pace of progress is going to be slow, but it can be steady. Don't get impatient and try to go through the entire progression in a month. Gradually "lowering" your starting position can pay huge dividends if you stick with it, and wait for your body to tell you it is time to make another change in the starting point.

Isometric Training

This type of training has largely been forgotten by lifting coaches for a variety of reasons. Thus, isometric training is probably completely unfamiliar to the current generation of lifters. However, there are huge potential benefits for power training.

Because the concept and practices are different from what is currently known, I have devoted a full chapter to isometric training, with demonstrations of how it could be incorporated into powerlifting training. This can be found in Chapter 11.

Chapter 10

Deadlift Training Cycles

In the next section, I'll present six different deadlift training cycles. Each one will include a specific amount of deadlifting, and assistance work that will help you build up your pulls.

It may seem obvious, but in order to perfect any of the powerlifts, deadlift included, it is necessary to practice them every week you train. A few *very experienced* lifters will emphasize training on assistance exercises to make gains. However, in my view, this strategy will work best only if you have been lifting for at least five years. Less experience than that, your key to success will be to work hard on each of the power lifts.

The five deadlift training cycles included here are organized with the deadlift sets coming first in the workout, followed by assistance exercises. I'm also assuming that you will be doing conditioning exercises at least every other training session.

You will do deadlifting **once a week.**

Each of the cycles introduces you to a new series of assistance exercises. You will probably find that you really like some of them, and absolutely hate others. Give all of them your best, and you will be properly rewarded:

1. Foundation cycle
2. Strength builder cycle
3. Band training
4. Power max cycle
5. Peaking cycle

If you are just starting out with power training, I suggest that you go through the cycles in the order above. If you are an experienced lifter, select any of the cycles that seem to meet your current needs. All of them will help you build a lot of power.

Remember; every cycle has a lot of benefits, but these will diminish rapidly, so you have to change your training every 4-8 weeks to continue to get stronger.

Recovery is really critical for improving in the deadlift. Very few top flight lifters train this lift more often than one time a week. A few lifts take a remarkable amount of energy.

For any lifter, recovery is the key to building big power and reaching your full potential. It is particularly important for lifters over age 50.

Deadlift Cycle #1 - Foundation Cycle

The foundation program for the deadlift is designed to build up your basic body strength and help develop outstanding technique. If you are new to powerlifting this is where you should begin your training. If you are an experienced lifter, you can use this routine over and over again to build up your strength.

This program will take a lot of energy, and it will take you a longer time to recover than you may realize. Thus you will only do this program **once a week.**

You should stay on this cycle for eight weeks. You will be amazed at how much stronger you have become after two months on this program.

The foundation program calls for the lifter to do 5 sets of 5 reps of the deadlift. You will use weights that are a percentage of your current 1 rep maximum lift. Each week, you will increase the weights in each set by 5 pounds (2.5 Kg).

That will be a 40-pound increase in each set over a two-month time period. It means that you will be lifting an additional of 250 pounds (115 Kg) each week as you progress through the cycle. That means that your work load on the final day of the cycle will be a half ton heavier than when you began.

I urge you not to get too aggressive on increasing the weight. This two-month cycle will be a challenge, and you don't want to have your progress plateau early by being too aggressive with weight increases.

Here is the deadlift foundation program:

Set 1: 50% of 1 rep max – 5 reps

Set 2: 60% of 1 rep max – 5 reps

Set 3: 75% of 1 rep max – 5 reps

Set 4: 80% of 1 rep max – 5 reps

Set 5: 60% of 1 rep max – 5 reps

When you have completed your 25 deadlifts, move on to your assistance work. In this stage of your training, your assistance work will be doing conditioning for deadlift training.

If you are an experienced lifter, you can use this 5 x 5 cycle to build more power. You can adjust the % of max lift upward 5% on two heavier sets. However, don't get too aggressive in the early going by using weight increases you can't sustain.

Assistance Work:

Kettlebell swing – Russian style

The kettlebells swing done Russian style can build huge power and resilience into your posterior power chain (aka the legs, butt and back).

The reason I refer to this as the "Russian" style swing is that there is a different version that is practiced in Cross Fit. The latter version has you extend the kettlebell overhead. This is a different exercise from the one I include here. Because both of these movements are called "the swing" considerable confusion arises over which swing we are discussing. You do the "Russian" version.

In this movement, begin in a standing position with feel shoulder width apart. Grasp the kettlebell (or dumbbell) with two hands with your arms hanging down in front of you. Bend your knees, and swing the bell back between your legs as if you were hiking a football. Keep your back flat and head erect.

You drive the kettlebell upward by quickly straightening your legs and throwing your hips forward. You do not apply any force with your arms. They are merely "ropes" that connect your body with the weight.

Drive the kettlebell to a position where your arms are parallel to the floor. Do not attempt to move the weight above this level. All of the force to move the kettlebell upward has come from driving your hips forward and straightening your legs.

If you are doing this movement properly, you will feel it in your abdominal muscles. If you feel it in your back, you are probably bent over or have a rounded back.

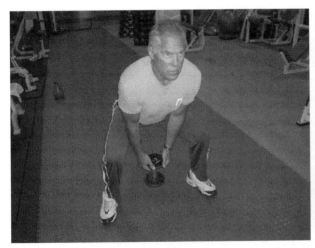 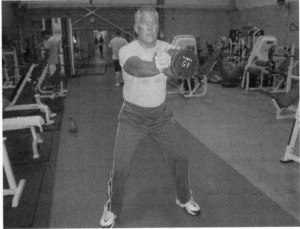

When the weight is at the top position, with your arms parallel to the floor, allow it to swing back down between your legs and repeat the motion of driving the weight upward with by quickly straightening your legs and driving your hips forward.

You should select a weight that gives you a challenge for 10 reps. Initially you will do 4 sets of 10. Each training session, you should try to add 2-3 reps to each set. By the end of 8 weeks you should be doing 4 sets of 20-25 reps each set.

The kettlebell handle is easy to grip with both hands. If you don't have access to heavier kettlebells, you can use dumbbells. In the photographs showing this exercise, the lifter is using a dumbbell. You can grip the dumbbell by the edges of the plates as shown, or place both hands on the handle.

The huge benefit of this exercise is that you will develop an armor plated back and abs. The Russian style swing is one of the greatest power builders ever developed. Practice it regularly and you will be rewarded with a bulletproof core.

In the foundation program, you will not be doing additional assistance work because the volume of lifting will be adequate to insure that you progress, but not so much that you become burned out or start falling back.

Both deadlifting and kettlebell/dumbbell swings take a lot out of you, and it is important that you are able to fully recover before your next training session.

If you feel compelled to do additional work, do hanging leg raises or other abdominal exercises.

You will also be doing the conditioning routine at the end of your workout. Needless to say, you can skip the kettlebell swings in that program if you have already done a large number in this program.

Deadlift Cycle #2 - Strength Builder Cycle

The deadlift builder program is an eight-week cycle where the workload increases significantly. Assistance work is ramped up and the lifter will work with more heavy weight on the deadlift.

Like all cycles, the specific poundage lifted in any given set is based on a percentage of the lifters 1 rep maximum lift. It is important that the number used in this calculation be the *current* one rep maximum, not some future target.

Like all the deadlift training cycles, you do this work out **once a week.**

Deadlifts in the cycle are as follows:

    Set 1: 60% of 1 rep max – 5 reps

    Set 2: 75% of 1 rep max – 3 reps

    Set 3: 80% of 1 rep max – 2 reps

    Set 4: 60% of 1 rep max – 5 reps

Increase the weight used by 5 pounds (2.5 Kg) each week. Insure that each and every deadlift is done from a *dead stop* off the floor. You get little benefit from merely touching the weight down and pulling it up. It is far more difficult to begin from a dead stop than from doing a "touch and go" pull.

You build big power by moving the weight from a dead stop. Remember, you want to win the competition, not the "workout".

Each week you add 5 pounds to the weight you used the week before. At the end of the cycle, you will have added 40 pounds to each set. Your total workload will be much higher than it was the first week, and your body strength will have increased significantly.

Assistance Work

Deadlift off Raised Surface

Lifting the deadlift bar from "below" the normal starting point is a huge strength builder. You need a small elevation to build big power in the lowest part of the pull. Usually 1" (3 cm) or 2" (6 cm) is sufficient to train your body to pull from "below" the usual starting point.

If you use any greater elevation, it will distort your form significantly and thus be of marginal utility to building big strength.

To get the most out of this movement, it is essential to Keep your back flat, shoulders back and body tense is critical in any deadlift movement. When you pull from below the normal starting point, you should feel the tension in your abs and not so much in your lower back.

As in all deadlift pulls, put upward tension on the bar before you actually pull it. Use the "over-under" deadlift grip…and plenty of chalk.

Begin your cycle with a weight that is 70% of your current 1 rep max. Start the cycle with 3 sets of 3 reps. Increase the weight by 5 pounds (2.5 Kg) every week for the first four weeks. At that point, do 3 sets of 2 reps and continue to increase the weight 5 pounds (2.5 Kg) for the remaining four weeks.

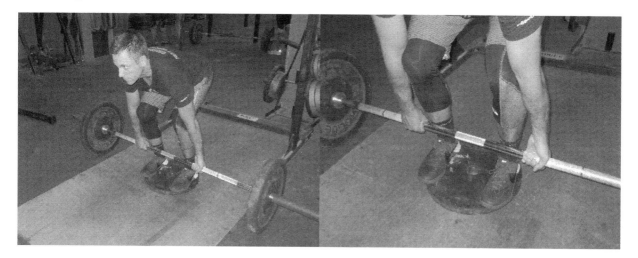

The purpose of this move is to train your body to put out a max effort at as high a speed as you can manage. Heavy weights may move slowly, but if you are moving them as fast as you can, you will be putting out 100% effort…maybe a bit more.

Remember…two sets….

Power rack partial deadlifts

Introducing partial deadlifts into your training is something that should be done with a bit of caution. If you have less than a year experience in power training, your body may not yet be able to support significant overloads that come with doing partial lifts. For this reason, I suggest that you go slow when you begin to do partial lifts.

The two versions of partial deadlifts are the one where the weight is set just below the knee, and the second where the bar is set just above the knee. When you begin doing these I would advise that you spend some time finding weights at both positions that give you a challenge, but don't over stress your back, neck and shoulders.

Eventually you will be able to do some huge weights when doing partial lifts, but in your first cycle, stay well below your 1 rep max for pulls below the knee, and don't go more than 5% over your 1 rep max for pulls above the knee.

Most people over age 50, even those who have been doing some weight training, will have some significant deficit in the strength of their back, neck and shoulders. It is critical when beginning power training that you recognize you must build up your baseload capacity in *all* parts of your back. If you have one weak link, it will cause problems.

The key is to *gradually* build the baseload strength needed to do really heavy training. This does not happen overnight. It happens by doing *consistent training* over weeks and months. It is far better to train conservatively and be able to train consistently than it is to be very aggressive and constantly have to deal with injuries. Those who are injured make little progress.

With that advice in mind, your first use of partial lifts should be limited to 2 sets of 2 reps at each rack height. Find weights you can handle with relative ease and increase them 5 pounds (2.5 Kg) each week during the cycle.

Experienced lifters can do 3-4 sets of a single rep at each height.

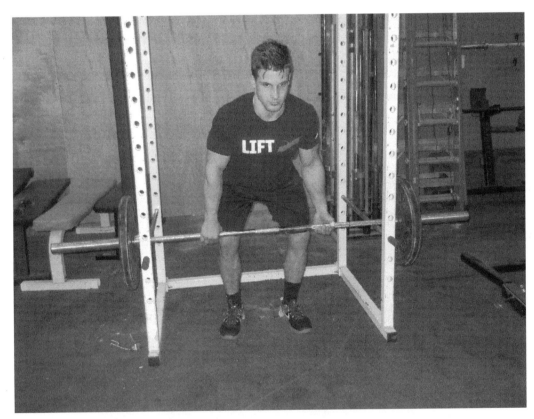

Starting position: set rack support pins to the desired height

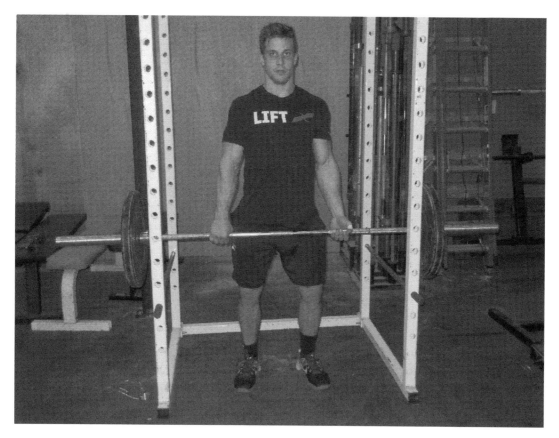

Finishing position: stand erect using perfect pulling form

You should finish off this workout with your conditioning training.

Deadlift Cycle #3 – Deadlift with Elastic Training Bands

This is a routine primarily when the lifter wants to build up base strength. There is a lot of volume, and some intriguing uses of rubberized bands to build up speed and overall power in the pull.

This is an eight-week cycle. It should be done **once a week.**

Each training session will involve slightly different combinations of sets and reps.

You will skip doing regular deadlifts since you will be doing the movement with some different variations in the five exercises in this program. Don't worry about not doing regular deadlifts, this cycle will give you all the work you want.

The first movement will employ elastic bands to alter the weight on the bar as you pull it. This creates unique tension in different phases of the lift.

Deadlifts with overhead bands

Do this exercise in a power cage. The lifting bar will be positioned on the floor in the middle of the power cage in position to do a deadlift.

Set a support rod on each side of the cage at approximately shoulder height. Loop an elastic exercise band around the midpoint of each support rod. The bottom of the band will loop around the lifting bar that will be set on the floor in position for the lifter to do a deadlift.

The easiest way to set this up is to attach the elastic bands to the support rods first, then place the lifting bar in the lower loops of the bands. The bands should be placed on the outside of the collars where the weights are loaded.

With the help of another person, load the first plates on to the lifting bar so that it goes down into position in the middle of the power cage. Once you have one heavy plate on the bar, it will be easy to load the others.

The purpose of this exercise is to pull a deadlift where the weight gets heavier as you get closer to the to the lockout. The elastic band will pull upward on the deadlift bar with anywhere from 35-60 pounds of tension when the bar is at the start position. As the lifter pulls the bar upward, the band tension on the bar eases, so that the weight being pulled *changes* as the bar comes up.

At the lockout position, there is little or no band tension on the bar. The lifter completes the last few inches to lockout holding the full weight of the bar.

Properly rigging the elastic bands on the lifting bar is very important. In the pictures below you see an example of how a deadlift bar is properly rigged.

You begin by attaching the elastic band to the top bar. In the picture the top bar is placed at roughly shoulder height. You may find that the tension the band puts on the bar is minimal at this height, so you will want to set the bar higher. The higher up you attach the band, the more tension and thus the more assist you get out of the bottom of the lift.

I would recommend that you begin attaching the bands to a bar that is just above the top of your head. You want a good boost out of the bottom of this lift, so err on the side of putting more tension on the bands rather than less.

Place the bands on the lifting bar on the side of the collar where you load the weights. This will prevent them from changing positions while you are lifting.

There are different sizes of elastic bands. The heavier bands provide more tension. The ones in the picture are medium weight. You should begin using light to medium bands. As you get stronger, you can use heavier bands.

Initially, load weight on the bar equal to 80% of your 1 rep max. Increase the weight on each of the five sets by 5-10 pounds. Your heaviest set should be the fourth of the five sets.

With the upward pull of the bands, the actual weight you pull off the floor will be quite a bit less. However, the weight being pulled as the bar comes up will get heavier as the bands relax.

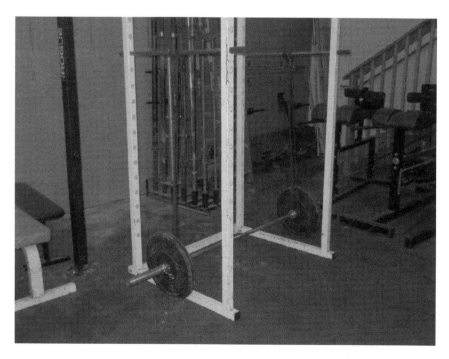

Elastic bands rigged to support max pull out of the bottom

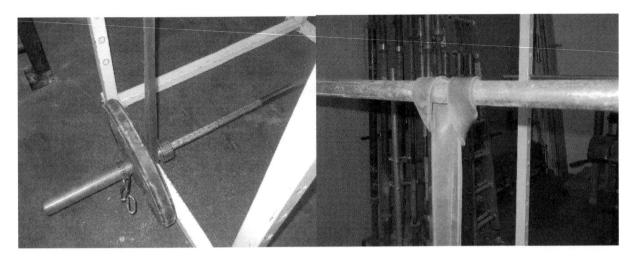

Proper way to secure elastic bands to deadlift bar

You will need to experiment to see how much weight you can pull with the bands giving you an assist out of the bottom. The reason I suggest experimenting is that there will be a difference in the strength of the bands.

This is an exhilarating exercise as over time you will wind up pulling quite a bit more weight than your current 1 rep max.

You should begin the cycle pulling your current 1 rep max in this lift. Add 5 pounds a week (or more if you feel strong). Do for **five sets of 2 reps.**

Each week add 5 pounds to each of your training sets.

Assistance Exercises

1. **Rumanian Deadlift**

One of the greatest training lifts ever devised, this is aimed strengthening your lower back, glutes and hamstrings.

Set up as if you were going to do a regular deadlift. Stand over the bar and take your normal grip. Take a deep breath and hold it, then *bend over at the waist with your legs slightly bent and your rear end up high. Keep your rear end up high and knees bent during the lift.*

Tense your body and put tension on the deadlift bar. Stand erect by pulling the bar up with your lower back, glutes and hamstrings.

Begin the cycle by pulling *about* 60% of your 1 rep max. You can increase the weight as you get stronger. This is one of those exercises where you need to feel your way along regarding weight increases. Many people, especially men, have relatively weak lower backs, and you should find weights that you can manage at the onset without risking injury.

You should aim for doing 3 sets of 3 reps in this exercise. Gradually increase the weight as you go through the cycle.

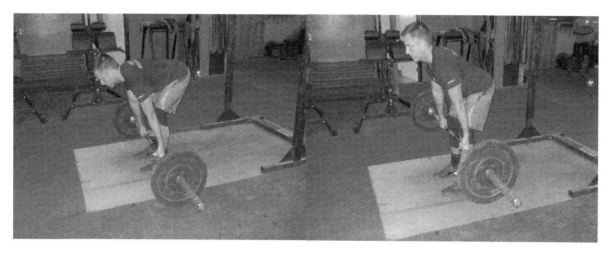

Beginning position   **Half way to lock out**

Partial Deadlift

The partial deadlift was developed mainly to assist squatters, but has great value for the deadlift as well. It will help build explosive strength in your glutes and hamstrings.

Unlike most assistance exercises, this one is to be done for *high reps* with light weights.

What do I mean by light weights?

Guys who deadlift over 700 pounds use a *maximum* of 225 pounds in this lift. The focus is on *explosiveness and speed,* not on grinding out heavy reps. Fifteen reps at a fast pace is the key to success. Oh yes…only do *two sets*…… (Note: when I say the number "two", this should not be interpreted to mean "5").

I have shown this move to a lot of lifters….and some of them immediately assumed that the "light weight" part of the advice did not apply to them. A week or two after showing them this quick explosive move, I would find them grinding 315 up and down….and quickly burning out…. At that point most of them would tell me that this exercise "sucked".

So much for detailed instructions….

If you deadlift 500 pounds or less, 165-185 is going to be as much as you want to use with this exercise.

This is one of those times when "more weight" should not be confused with "better"....

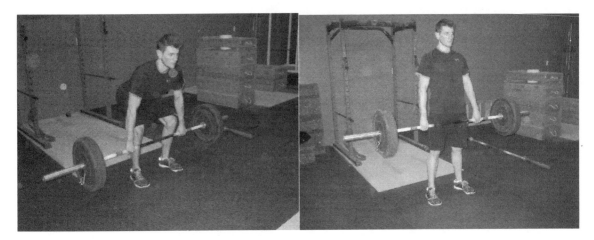

Starting position **Low position: don't put weigh on floor**

Think of this as "speed work" for the deadlift. You begin by gripping the bar with both hands being palms in (power clean grip). Get in your starting position for the deadlift, and raise the bar to halfway up your shins. This is the starting point.

When the bar is motionless halfway up you shins, you quickly stand erect in a full deadlift lockout position. You stand erect as fast as you can move the bar. Drive your hips forward explosively as the bar clears your knees.

Do a full legal lock out with head erect and shoulders back. Then instantly drop the bar back to the starting point halfway up your shins.

Each time you stand fully erect, you immediately drop the bar back to the midpoint of your shins and immediately accelerate upward at full speed.

You *never* allow the bar to touch the floor or bounce upward in any way.

If you are moving the weight as fast as you can (under control) you will find that 15 reps with a "light" weight is a pretty serious effort. Do two sets.

Leg Press

Despite my general dislike of machine exercises, the leg press can be useful as an assistance exercise for the deadlift. It is important that you use the leg press to simulate the leg position you will have when you pull the weight off the floor.

The leg press can give your quadriceps more strength for "pushing into the floor" in the initial pull off the floor. If you do the leg press with the intent of feeling the quads "push" the weight into the floor, you can further add to your deadlifting power.

Find a weight that you can do for 3 sets of 5 reps and gradually increase it over time. It is critical that you do deep leg presses that simulate the angle your quads will be at when you deadlift. It is worthless to do presses where you barely bend the leg.

Deadlift Cycle #4 - Power Max Cycle

This cycle is an eight-week program that you use to prepare for a peaking cycle, or do in the off season when you want to boost your personal best.

In this program you will do deadlifts 7 sets of 2 reps each with progressively heavier weights until the 5th set. Following that you will do assistance work that begins the deadlift from a lower starting position than normal.

The cycle is as follows:

Set 1: 55% of 1 rep max – 2 reps

Set 2: 70% of 1 rep max – 2 reps

Set 3: 75% of 1 rep max – 2 reps

Set 4: 80% of 1 rep max – 2 reps

Set 5: 85% of 1 rep max – 2 reps

Set 6: 70% of 1 rep max – 2 reps

Set 7: 55% of 1 rep max- 2 reps

As always, use perfect technique and do each rep from a complete dead stop.

Add 5 pounds to the first four sets every week. Add 5 pounds to set 5 every two weeks. Do not add weight to sets 6 and 7.

Assistance Exercises

Deadlift off a raised surface

One of the movements that helps you get the weight started off the floor is to deadlift with your feet on a low block. This creates the effect of starting to pull the bar below normal bar height.

The block need only be 2" or 3" in height. Anything higher distorts your form so much that the training benefit is reduced.

As you can see in the photograph, you can use a 45 lb barbell plate for your "elevation". You don't want to pull from too great a height, because it distorts your lifting form. Besides, you get most of the benefit from lifting off an elevated platform from the first inch or two.

Going below the normal starting position will help develop power for the start of the lift when you are fighting to overcome the forces of gravity and inertia. The rule in physics that says "a body at rest tends to remain at rest" is will never be clearer to you than when you begin to pull on a deadlift bar.

Deadlifting from a little below the normal starting point can help you be better prepared to overcome the forces of gravity…..

Do 3 sets of 3 reps with this beginning with a weight you can pull relatively easily. Increase the weight on each set.

Rumanian Deadlift

If the good morning exercise looked like a bad squat, the Rumanian Deadlift looks like a poorly done straight leg deadlift. In reality, this is one of the greatest builders of lower back strength ever devised.

Load the bar as if you were going to do a regular deadlift. When you stand over the bar, your shins will be against the bar and your feet in position for a conventional deadlift.

Bend over and grip the bar, keeping your back flat, with your knees slightly bent, and your tail end elevated….or "way up in the air".

Pull the bar off the floor and stand erect. Your knees should be flexed during the pull, *not straight*. It is really important that your back be flat during the pull.

This will really tax your lower back. That is the purpose of the lift.

You will want to do 3 sets of 3 reps with a reasonably demanding weight. You will build super back strength, and go a long way toward protecting yourself against injury.

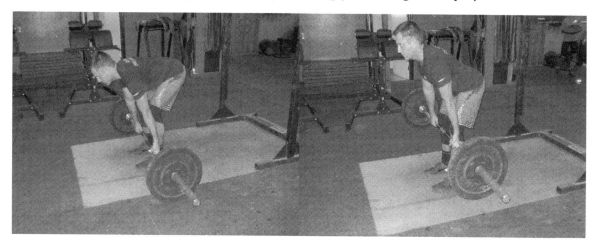

Deadlift Cycle #5 - Short Peaking Cycle

This training cycle is one you should use when you are preparing for a contest, or training to set (but not at) your limit.

For this reason, you should be very careful not to overdo the heavy work. If some lift feels too heavy on a given day, *don't do it!* You will make a lot more progress if you recognize that some days you will not have recovered sufficiently to do the heavy pulls you had planned. Toughing it out when you feel like crap may make you feel like you overcame fatigue, but it will cost you big time in the coming weeks.

Forcing heavy reps during a peaking cycle can also lead to serious, occasionally catastrophic, injury. I know lifters who suffered injuries that required surgery and had them in rehab for six months to a year because they forced their bodies to do something that their body was (demonstrably) not able to do.

I'll harp on the idea that you are training for your own fitness, and with the intention of winning the contest, not "winning the workout". If you are over age 50, you can accomplish mind blowing lifts, *but* you can't do this without listening to your body when it tells you that you may not be up to pulling a certain weight in a heavy workout.

This is true for people under 50…and under 40 and in their 20's. Keep in mind that a lot of sensational lifts were "left in the gym" because the person training didn't know when to push and when to take a rest.

With that caveat, let's look at the 4 week peaking cycle. The contest will occur the week following the fourth week of the cycle.

As I noted earlier, I believe that short peaking cycles can be extremely effective if you have a good base of conditioning.

You will do this work out **_once a week_** during the peaking period. You will be aiming to increase your best deadlift by 3-5%. If you have been competing for a while, that will be a significant increase.

You will use your *current* one rep maximum as the basis for calculating the weights you will lift during each work out.

Week 1:

    Set 1: 60% - 3 reps

    Set 2: 75% - 2 reps

    Set 3: 80% - 2 reps

Set 4: 80% - 1 rep

Assistance exercise

Week 2:

Set 1: 65% - 3 reps

Set 2: 75% - 2 reps

Set 3: 85% - 1 rep

Set 4: 90% - 1 rep

Assistance Exercise

Week 3:

Set 1: 65% - 3 reps

Set 2: 80% - 2 reps

Set 3: 95% - 1 rep

Assistance Exercise

Week 4:

Set 1: 65% - 1 rep

Set 2: 85% - 1 rep

Set 3: 98% - 1 rep

No assistance work

Week 5: The Contest

1st Attempt – 95% of 1 rep max

2nd Attempt – 1 rep max + 5 lbs (2.5 Kg)

3rd Attempt – 103-105% of 1 rep max

Assistance Work

In this cycle, you will use assistance work in the first three weeks of the program, and eliminate it in the fourth week. The purpose is to conserve your energy for your contest attempts.

Power Cage lockouts

Do two sets of one rep at the position just below the knees, and two sets of a single rep at the position above the knees.

Below the knees, use weights that require about a 90% exertion. Above the knees aim for weights that are at least 100 lbs (50 Kg) above the weight you will use in your full deadlift.

Deadlifts off a raised surface

Do two sets of two reps while standing on a block or barbell plate that is about 1-inch-high (3 cm). Do not use a raised platform that is any higher than this. Your primary objective is to put the finishing touches on your pull off the floor. Using a higher elevation raised surface a month before a PR attempt will actually hinder your chances of succeeding.

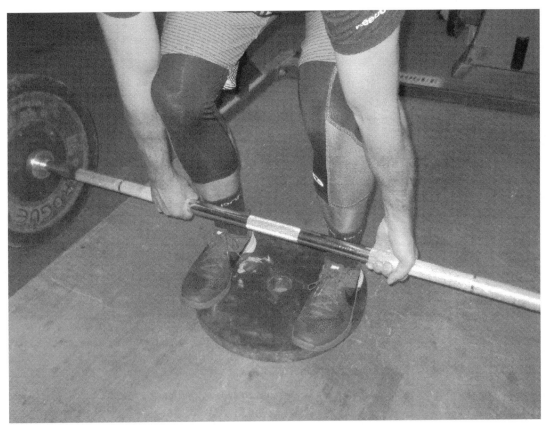

Kettlebell swing

Complete your assistance work with 3 sets of 10-20 heavy kettlebell swings.

The final week before the contest or max attempt you should train with *very light* weights and do nothing more than break a sweat. If you are planning on deadlifting 500 lbs in the contest, you should do no more than 135 lbs in the final week. Just remind your body of how the lift is done.

You can do *light* athletic activity, such as shooting baskets (*not* playing full court basketball), light yoga, or jogging. Don't do intense activity.

You should use a therapeutic sauna if it is available to you. Steam baths and whirlpools are also good if available. In no event should you cook yourself or try some "sweat lodge" treatment. You need to build your strength and energy for the contest.

Additional Deadlift Assistance Exercises

The following group of exercises are considered "advanced" in part because they require special pieces of equipment nor available in most gyms, and in part because at least one of them is extraordinarily difficult to do.

Reverse Hyperextension

This movement can add a lot to your back strength, but it requires a piece of equipment that is not found in most gyms.

The "reverse hyper" machine works the lower back in ways that nothing else can. It both strengthens and stretches the muscles around your spinal cord, while building and stretching your hamstrings and glutes.

You lie on your stomach on the platform with your legs hanging straight down and your feet hooked inside the strap attached to the weight arm. Grab the handles to make certain you don't slide off the machine. You should begin using a light weight, and work up as you are able to get stronger.

Begin by swinging your legs back and up so that you finish the upward movement with your legs out straight. This will require a strong contraction in your lower back, abs, glutes and hamstrings.

When you are at the top of the contraction, relax and allow the weight to pull your legs down. Then swing your legs forward under the platform. This will stretch your back muscles and elongate your spine. Then drive your legs upward again until your muscles are fully contracted.

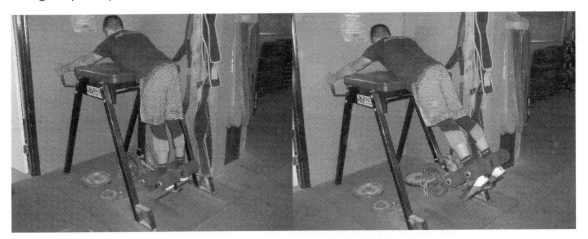

Starting position **Pulling upward**

The movement will be a rhythmic swing from the top position to the bottom and back up. Allow the momentum to move the weight and move your lower back through a range from contraction to stretching. It should feel good.

Begin by doing 3 sets of 10 reps and gradually build up the weight you use. In this exercise the weight is less important than completing the full range of motion of the leg swing.

Back Hyperextensions

The back hyperextension chair is widely available in gyms, so this is an exercise that you can do just about everywhere.

Place your hips on the seat while lying face down, and secure your feet in the restraining stirrups.

Begin with your upper body extended and parallel to the floor. You will bend forward until your upper body is at a right angle to the floor. At this point, raise yourself back to the starting position.

The effort of raising your upper body back to the start point is done by your lower back, glutes, abs and hamstrings.

To make this movement more challenging, you can hold a barbell plate against your chest.

You should do this exercise for 3 sets of 10 reps. Over time you should add weight so that it is a continuing challenge.

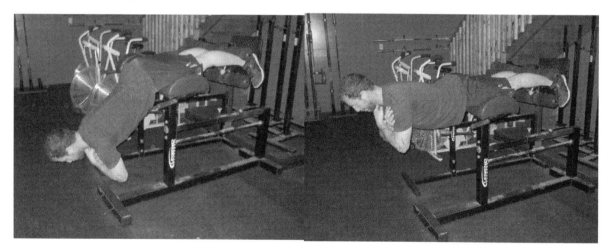

Lower your body to this point or below   **Raise up to this position**

Spinal Erector Band Pulls

This movement develops an explosive pull in the deadlift. It is one of those movements that is great for a mini-cycle. Thus, you will practice this for about four weeks at a time, two to four times a year.

Attach an elastic band to a well anchored support. When you pull on the band, you will pull hard on the support, so it had better not move or you could be in trouble.

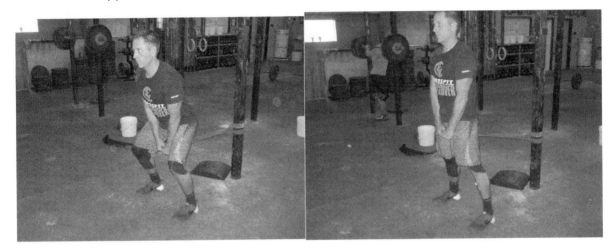

Start: hold band firmly   **Drive upright with explosive movement**

When you have the band attached, place the band between your legs and hold the free end with both hands. Your hands will be holding the band between your legs.

Bend over and allow your hands holding the band to go back as if you were going to hike a football. Take a few steps away from the support so that the band gets somewhat tight.

To perform the exercise, rapidly drive your chest and shoulders to an erect position. The band will strongly resist this movement, and you may lose your balance. You need to steady yourself, return to the bent over position again rapidly drive your chest and shoulders to the erect position.

You should feel a strong sensation in your abs, glutes and hamstrings.

You should do 10-15 reps of this movement for 2-3 sets.

Note: You can also do a version of this lift using the cable row machine. Grasp the handle that is connected to the weight stack and pull it as shown above.

Chapter 11

Isometrics: A Forgotten Training Method that Promotes Big Gains

With a title like that, most of you will either skip the chapter entirely, or go immediately to the exercises. Actually, the training method is not so much a secret, as it is forgotten.

Let me begin back in 1960 when I was doing Olympic Style lifting while I was a student at Michigan State. Our coach (the late legendary Pat O'Shea) was friends with the top lifters in the US and some other parts of the world. In the 1960 World Championships, the Polish team had surprised everyone by dominating the competition where they had been secondary players before.

It turned out that they had devised a completely new training protocol that was really different from the way everyone else trained. It was called "Isometrics".

Basically what the training did was break down the competitive lift into increments of 1-2 inches (3-6 cm). Then the trainee would exert full force against a static resistance set every 1-2 inches through the full range of the lift.

The trainee would be standing in a power cage where they would pull (or push) a lifting bar using the maximum force their body could generate against immovable restraining pins set at different heights. The idea was to duplicate the full range of a given lift, and allow the trainee to experience putting out maximum force at every point in the lift.

For example, to replicate the power clean, the beginning position of the bar was at the height where the bar would be when resting on the floor. The next position would be an inch or two higher. The progression up the power cage would continue through the full range of the lift.

At each point, the trainee pulled as hard as they could against a pin that prevented the lifting bar from moving. The objective was to train the body to put out maximum force for a few seconds at whatever height the bar was positioned.

Since the purpose of the static bar was to duplicate the full range of an Olympic lift, the bar position was changed after each push or pull. Starting with the lifting bar on the floor, the restraints were gradually raised through the full range of a clean, press, jerk, or snatch.

The reason this training was so effective is that there are points throughout the full lift where lifters are weaker or stronger. When doing the full lift, the momentum generated in a strong portion of the lift can move the bar through those places where lifters are weaker. Because the bar is moving rapidly, it is impossible to train the weak points in isolation.

Isometric training allowed coaches to isolate those places in an individual lift where a lifter was weaker, and strengthen those.

Weak points in a lift are often called "sticking points". These are often where the work of lifting is changing from one group of muscles to another. Weak points can also be where a lifter has not trained their body to put out maximal force.

For either of these situations, strengthening weak points meant a better overall lift.

Another benefit of using isometrics was that the lifters *overall strength* made a significant jump. Apparently working against a bar that cannot move allowed each lifter to build greater strength capacity at individual points in the lift. When the bar is moving this is impossible because the bar will quickly move through each point in the lift.

Some fifty years later, I'm suggesting that you can benefit from integrating a simplified version of this training into your own program for getting stronger. What I will present below are isometric training workouts for the squat, bench press and deadlift.

Isometric training has one unique strength building benefit that is nearly impossible to train any other way. That is teaching your body to put out *maximum power* at different points in a lift. This is done by pulling a weight from a set position against a stationary restraining rod. The lifter pulls with maximum force against the stationary rod. The restraining rod won't move, but the lifter is able to try to move the immovable by putting out the greatest amount of force they can.

Over time, the lifter adapts to the static training by developing the ability to put out greater amounts of force than they could when the bar was moving fast.

Isometrics and Power Training

Isometric training has been largely ignored by powerlifting coaches. The reasons are not too hard to understand. Isometric movements are very unusual for weight training. Most people only involve moving the weight bar a few inches at any one time.

The original isometric protocol called for lifters to do isometric training six days a week. However, during this period the lifters did *no other type of weight training.* There are not many lifters I know who could do this routine without going nuts.

One of the real joys of doing physical training is the feeling of *movement.* In the original protocol stressed building power with isometrics, and proper technique in Olympic style lifting by doing literally hundreds of reps with a broomstick (no weight) to get the form of the competition lift perfect.

However, I believe isometric training has the potential to significantly improve any lifters performance if included on a regular basis in training cycles as assistance work.

The huge advantage of isometric training is the ability to generate big overloads *at specific points in the lift*. This will enable you to build maximum power in some parts of the lift where you may be weak or have a sticking point.

All isometric training is done in a power rack. The bar will rest on one set of pins, with another set of pins 2-3" above. The isometric lift consists of driving the bar upward until it is stopped by the second (restraining) pins. At that point, you exert *maximum force* for roughly 5 seconds before lowering the bar to the starting position. To make it simple, I suggest that during the period of maximum exertion, you "count to five" in your head.

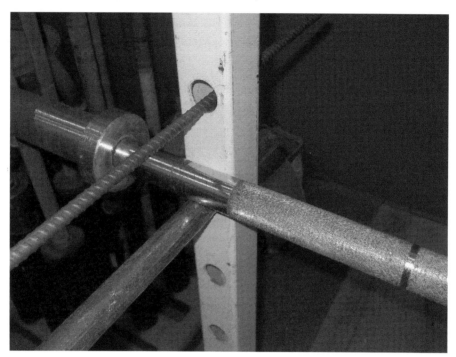

In the picture you see the lifting bar resting on the support pin, and the restraining pin positioned just above it. The support pins are the strong rods that are in the power rack to support heavy weights. The restraining pins can be a simple piece of rebar which can be purchased at a building supply company.

Few lifters have any experience of generating maximum force. They typical gym lifter will usually put out 50-70% of their maximum force potential during their regular training. Powerlifters put out a considerably higher percentage of their maximum potential. The purpose of isometrics for a powerlifter is to *train* your body to put out maximum force *and* do exercises that *increase* the actual amount of force you can generate.

Isometrics is a great way to both teach your body put all the force you can into a single rep, and be able to increase to amount of force you can generate. The cool thing is that isometrics allow you to work on building force generating capacity at *discreet parts of the lift*.

Putting out full power should never be confused with "training to failure". Doing a lot of reps until you can't do any more is an endurance issue, not a power issue. High rep sets rarely use weights that are heavier than 60-70% of one rep max.

In isometrics, the idea is to generate 100-110% of the force you would normally be able to generate at a specific point in a lift. If the weight is moving, the upward momentum of the bar will contribute to moving past a sticking point. By placing a restraining rod at a certain point in the lift, it becomes impossible to generate any momentum. All the pulling will be from a static position.

A word of caution. You must be certain that *the cage* you are using will not move when you pull upward against the pins. Many power cages are bolted to the gym floor. If this is the case, you should have no problem. If they are not bolted to the floor, you will need to make certain that they will not move when you lift the barbell up against the pins.

The program I'll lay out here will give you the basics of using isometric training.

You can use isometrics as part of your assistance exercise for any of the lifts. Ideally, you should do isometrics twice a week. You can even do them three times a week. Do your isometric training for 4-weeks at a time. Take a break for a few weeks and come back to it if you desire.

Isometric training for the Squat

I'll show three different positions for doing isometrics to train the squat. They come at different heights in the squat, and target the points where most people have difficulty.

Below Parallel

This is the most difficult position for most lifters when doing competition squats. Going below parallel with a heavy weight is hugely stressful both physically and mentally. Doing some isometric sets can help build confidence and strength.

Begin by setting the lower pin at a position where you can take the bar on your back as if you had done a full squat. This may take some experimenting, and you may find it is difficult to get under a bar that is very low. However, if you are persistent, you will soon develop the flexibility and agility to get into proper position.

You should be using a *very light* weight on this. Begin by using no added weight on the bar. The issue will not be how much you can move from the deep bottom, but how much force you can generate when pushing against the restraining pins.

Arrange the bar so that it is on your back the same way it would be in a regular competition squat. Then adjust yourself so that you are in exactly the same form you are supposed to be in when at the bottom of a deep squat. That is chest up, tail down, back flat and head erect.

You will need to get really tight down in the cramped starting position. This is essential to mobilize maximum force, and to protect your back, knees, legs, etc.

When you have the bar properly positioned on your back, and you have assumed proper body alignment, take a deep breath and hold it. Then push the weight up until the lifting bar contacts the restraining pin above. The restraining pin should be set at a point where you would be just below parallel.

When you contact the restraining pin, keep your body aligned in perfect form and begin to press upward as hard as you can *without compromising your form.* Keep your chest up and your tail end down. When the lifting bar contacts the upper pin, push as hard as you can against the pin for a count of five. Then release your breath and lower the bar back to the starting position.

If it is a question of keeping good form, or pressing upward with all your might, concentrate on to keeping good form. You will get a lot of benefit from this. If you start pushing upward and allow your butt to come up, or alter your leg drive, you are defeating the purpose of the exercise.

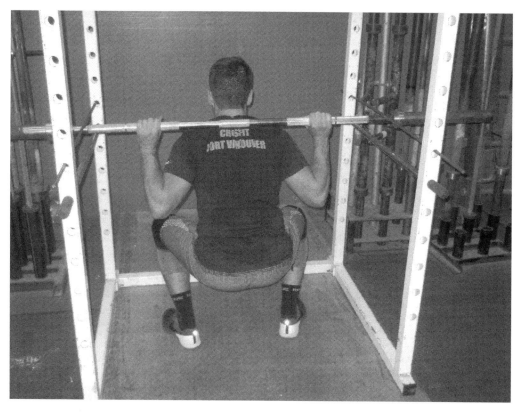

Isometric rack positioned for training the low portion of the squat

You will be doing this **2 times for a count of 5**. When you have done the first push, relax and set the weight back on the bottom pins. If you wish, you can step out of the cage for a minute or two. If you would prefer, you can wait 30-60 seconds in the deep squat position, and then do your second push.

The position below parallel is very unusual and uncomfortable. It may take you quite a while to master getting into it, and doing the movement with good technique. Keep practicing and you will be rewarded many times over.

Just above parallel

The second setting for squat isometrics is a few inches *above* parallel. You can adjust the pins on the power cage to raise the bottom support so that you can get under the lifting bar more easily than in the low squat position.

Just above parallel is where many lifters lose their squats because it is at this point that you change from one set of muscles providing the main push to another. This transition area is often called the "sticking point".

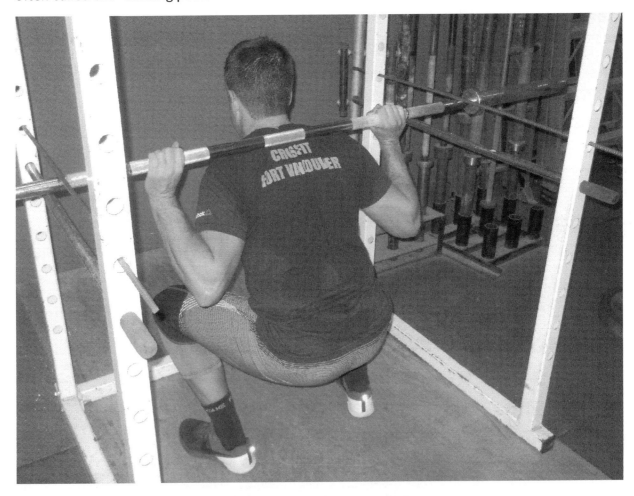

Position just above parallel

Like the deep squat isometric, you must have perfect technique and be completely tight during the push. You will also use a light weight.

The biggest threat to not having perfect form is the inclination for your butt to raise up during the maximum push. The "tail up first" movement is one of the most common errors in coming out of the bottom of a deep squat. If you practice perfect form in your isometric training, it will be much easier to prevent this flaw from coming into your squatting.

As before, you will exert maximum force upward for a count of five, then relax. Take a 30-60 second rest and repeat the exertion. Again, you will only do **two** pushes at this level.

Partially erect

The third and final position for doing isometric squats will be the position you will be in when you are about 2/3 of the way up from the bottom.

Adjust the lower pin so that you can take the weight about 2" below where you will push against the restraining bar. You should load the bar to roughly 30% of your 1 rep max lift. A light weight, but one that is substantial enough to insure that you have to work to control it.

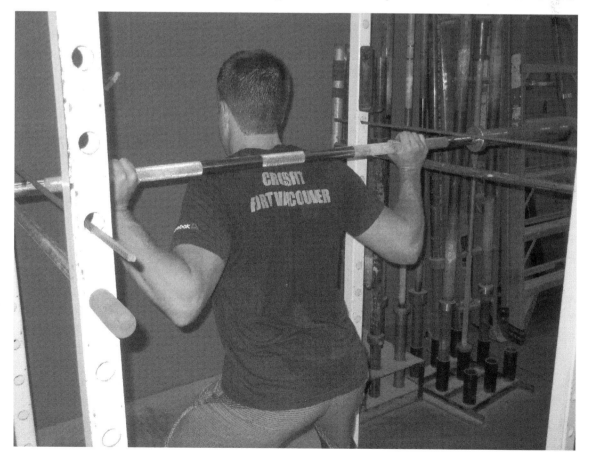

Partially erect position

Make certain that the weight is properly positioned on your back, insure you have proper body alignment for perfect form, take a deep breath and hold it, then push the weight up until it contacts the restraining pin.

The important thing about this exercise is that you train yourself to exert maximum force using perfect form. Keep the chest up and your tail end down. Keep your back flat and never allow yourself to roll forward.

Push hard against the restraining bar for a count of five. Then relax and lower the weight to the starting position. As before, do **2 five count pushes.**

Having done a total of 6 maximum exertion pushes against an immovable bar, you will have done a lot of work. The exertion may not sound like a lot when you read it, but the actual amount of effort is truly formidable.

Isometrics for the Bench Press

Isometric training on the bench press is particularly useful for building power to blast through the dreaded "sticking points". Isometrics can also help the lockout portion of the lift.

The three points to set the pins at are:

- Just off the chest
- 3 inches (10 cm) above the chest
- 2 inches (7 cm) below full lock out

Just off the chest

When a pause is introduced into bench pressing, the first real difficulty emerges is the initial push off the chest. Doing isometric training at this portion of the lift can improve both the stability of the bar on the chest, but also the first upward push off the chest.

You will lift from a bench that can be positioned in the middle of the power cage as shown in the photographs. This bench should be the same height as a competition bench. This is important because you want to use the same body alignment on this bench as you would on a regular competition bench.

Begin by setting the pin that will support the weight *slightly below* where the bar would rest on your chest. Since the bar will be *lower* than the starting point in the lift, you will have to begin this lift by adjusting the bar on your chest as if it were in the pause position.

Set the restraining (top) pin at a point where it will stop the lifting bar just above your chest.

You will use a light weight or even an empty bar on this exercise since the principal benefit will be the intense contraction when you press the bar against the restraining pin just off the chest.

Position yourself on the bench as if you were going to do a competition lift. Insure that your feet, back and shoulders are positioned exactly the same way as they would if you were going to attempt a maximum single lift. Your entire body will be tight.

Position the lifting bar on your chest as if it were a super heavy weight. You will be driving your shoulders toward your toes and tensing your entire body. Dig your feet into the floor, and press the bar upward until it is stopped by the restraining pin.

You should push with all your strength against the restraining pin for a count of five, then relax and allow the bar to return to your chest.

Rest for 30 seconds or so, and repeat. As in the other lifts, you will do **2 intense contractions.**

Then it is time to raise the bar to the next height to continue the training session.

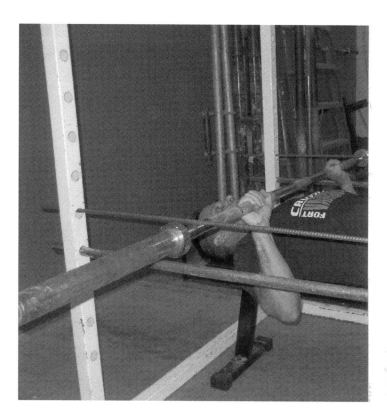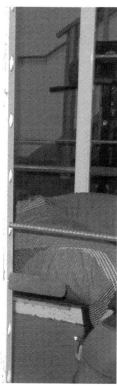

Isometric push from the chest

Just above the chest

Set the restraining pin so that the upward movement of the bar will be stopped roughly 3 inches (10 cm) above your chest. This is usually where a major sticking point occurs in the bench press. This will usually be only one hole higher on the power rack support settings.

Set the support pins so that you begin the lift an inch or so off your chest. You should use a very light weight or an empty bar for this exercise.

As before, position yourself on the bench, get completely tight, and drive the bar off the support pin into the restraining pin. Keeping perfect form, push as hard as it is possible for you to push for a count of five. Then relax and allow the bar to go back to the lower pin.

After a 30-60 second rest, do your second intense contraction.

Then, raise the bar to the final position you will use in your bench press isometric training.

Just below full lock out

Often completing the full lock out is difficult when bench pressing a big weight. The third position in the bench isometric program calls for you to set the restraining bar just below your own lock out position.

Set the restraining (upper) pin so that your elbows are not fully extended. Ideally, this would be about 1-2 inches (3-7 cm) below the point where your elbows are completely straight in a full lock out.

The support pin (lower) should be set roughly 2 inches (7 cm) below the restraining pin.

You should use a relatively light weight on this lift, but since you will be pushing the weight almost at arm's length, you can use 50-60% of your 1 rep max. The key thing is that you will be exerting as much force as you can generate against the restraining pin.

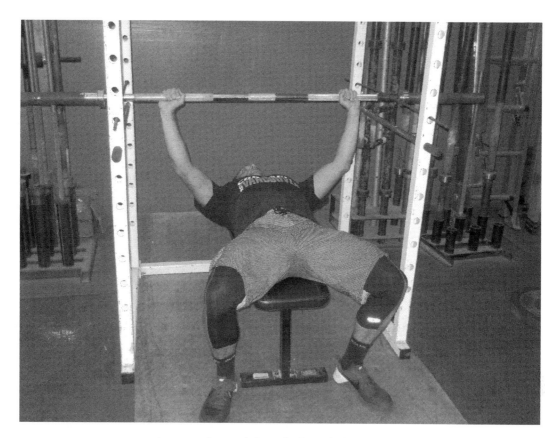

Isometric push just below full lock out

As in the other isometric lifts, you will use perfect technique and exert maximum force against the restraining pin for a count of five. Do 2 of these intense contractions.

Isometrics for Deadlift

Initial Pull

The initial pull off the floor is one of the places where isometric training can really give you a big boost. This begins with the barbell on the floor with you standing inside the power rack as shown. The barbell plates should be competition diameter so that you start the pull at the normal height. Set the pin that will stop the bar's upward movement at 1" or less above where the bar is sitting on the floor.

What you are doing here is setting the bar at the starting point, and setting the restraining pins so that you will be pulling as hard as you can against an immovable object.

Load the bar to 50% of your 1 rep max. Stand and grip the bar as if you were doing a contest deadlift. Pull the bar up with maximal force until it is stopped by the pin. Hold it against the restraining pin for 3-5 seconds while pulling as hard as you can.

You must use *perfect form*. If you are pulling differently than you would with a regular deadlift, the training effect will be minimal.

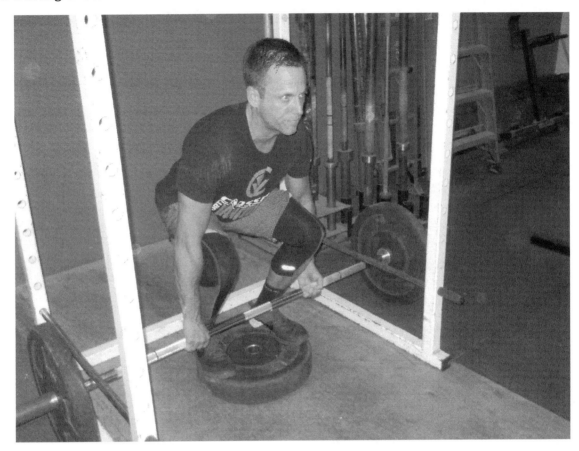

Pulling from the start position

You should also go through the process of "getting tight" before you pull the bar. You want the isometric pull to be exactly like you would pull in a contest…except the bar is stopped by the restraining pin.

For the initial pull, you want the restraining pin to stop the upward movement of the bar at (or very slightly below) the point where you would begin your deadlift. To position yourself at this point, you may have to stand on barbell plates or plywood panels to be in proper position.

In the picture the lifter is standing on a barbell plate. This is because the lowest hole in the power rack is too high to be positioned to restrict the pull at the very start of the lift. Depending on how your power rack is built, you may have to improvise like this.

1. Below the Knee

Set the upper (restraining) rod at the point where you want the bar to stop. Set the lower rod 2-3" below the upper rod. Here is where the barbell will rest when you begin your pull.

Use a barbell loaded to about 50% of your one rep max. It will rest on the lower of the two rods.

Set up so that you are completely tight, and are in the exact position you should be when the upward movement of the bar is stopped by the restraining rod. Grip the bar, pull your shoulders back, and pull the bar up until it touches the restraining rod. Pull as hard as it is possible for you to pull for about 3 seconds. The bar is immovable, but you are pulling as hard as your body can to pull trying to drive it "through" the restraining rod.

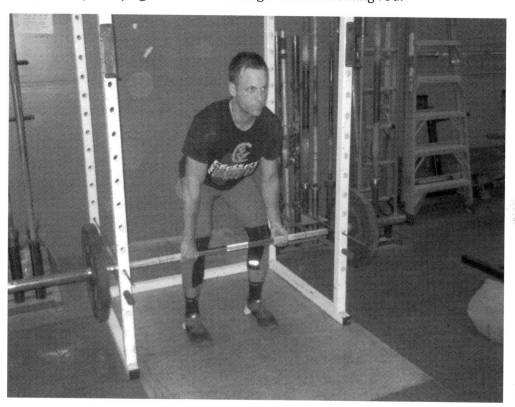

Pulling just below the knee

Pulling against this immovable barrier for 3-5 seconds will train your central nervous system to put out massive force at specific parts of the lift. This training will make you stronger because not only will your muscle fibers be forced to grow, but your central nervous system will be trained to put out maximum force.

2. **Above the knee**

Set the lower rod at the position where you want to begin the pull. Set the restraining rod 2-3" above the lower rod. Load the bar to roughly 60-70% of your one rep maximum. Now repeat the process of getting tight and duplicating the form you should be using at that portion of your pull.

As before, pull the bar as hard as you can against the restraining rod for a count of five. Then lower the bar back to the support rod. Perfect technique is mandatory.

It is critical not to do too much isometric training because the central nervous system and your muscles can be over stressed by too much overload. You get the most benefit from doing a *total* of 3-6 total isometric pulls. Anything beyond that, and you will be going backwards.

Remember, the way to build strength is to lift heavy weights *and recover!*

Now a mandatory safety warning. When you pull upward on any power cage, you have the potential to flip it over or create an otherwise dangerous situation. Insure that the cage you are using *will not move or fall over* when you are pulling upward with maximum force.

The first thing to do is check and see if the cage you plan to use is bolted to the floor. Many are not bolted down, since some gyms want to move them around for different uses.

Securing the power cage to the floor is critical if you don't want an accident. If the cage is light and not bolted to the floor, you can use heavy dumbbells (or sand bags) placed on the base to keep the whole cage from moving. You may have to get creative on how you arrange the dumbbells, but generally you can find a way to keep almost any power cage in place while you pull upward against the restraining rods.

Make *absolutely* certain you can't tip over the cage during your isometric pulling session. Don't be lazy about securing the cage.

You should regard the work of hauling heavy dumbbells to the cage to prevent any movement as part of your training. Strong people haul lots of "heavy stuff" as part of life. The pencil necks have their personal trainer load the bar for them to do arm curls, and the bar must be set in a squat cage so they don't have to bend over to pick it up.

Part III
More Very Important Information:
Getting the most out of your life in the gym

Food for thought:

"The unexamined life is not worth living."

-Socrates

"Each man must accept the cards life deals him. But, once they are in hand, he alone must decide how to play the cards in order to win the game"

- Voltaire

Chapter 12

The Pathway to Success: Small Steps to Big Improvements

If your objective is to become the best lifter you can be, you should *immediately* begin thinking about your training in a different light than perhaps you did before. From now on, everything you do in training is purposefully designed to help you improve. Your sole purpose of doing <u>any</u> training session or workout <u>*is to improve your capabilities as a powerlifter*</u>.

What this means is that *whenever you train,* you will be doing one or more of the following: 1) improve athletic skill; 2) building your power or; 3) improving some mental capability that will contribute to your success. Most of the time, you will be working on all three simultaneously.

It is important that you *explicitly* recognize what you are doing each time you practice or train. For example, if you are doing single rep deadlifts you should be training on your maximum power output, perfect form, and the mental focus needed to put maximum effort into a lift. If you are doing bench presses with elastic bands attached to the bar, you will be working on mobilizing all of the support muscles in your body when you do the lift.

Never train without an explicit purpose. Everything you do should use your time, energy and focus to the greatest efficiency.

Your entire mental focus should be on what <u>you</u> are doing and what <u>you</u> intend to do. Don't get mentally involved with what anyone else in the gym is doing (with the exception of those who are training with you). Other people's lack of direction is not your problem. Looking at others and thinking about what they are doing is a total waste of your mental energy.

When you adopt this attitude, your outward behavior during training will just be of someone going about their business. You have a job to do, and you are doing it. All of your energy and focus should be on *what <u>you</u> are doing,* and not on extraneous distractions.

After spending six decades in a variety of gyms, it seems to me that it is best to think of a gym as if it were a big cafeteria with lots of different buffet offerings. Everyone wants something different, and all can find something that suits them.

Only a *tiny* minority of people lifting in any gym will even be *interested* in doing power training. Most are there to be fit, be healthy, look good, and perhaps improve their performance in a sport totally different than power lifting. They are there for their own reasons, and you are there for yours. But, everyone gets to play with the toys.

Enough about "them", now let's focus on you, and how you go about your business.

The Biggest Factors in Success

Years ago I read an article written by a big time fitness consultant who asked the simple question "what are the most important factors in achieving success in the gym?" I won't make you guess, but there are two parts to the answer.

The first is having a _burning desire_ to achieve something.

Without having a powerful desire to achieve something, you will never get past the first week of training. It is critical to understand that the term *burning desire* does not mean, "if it isn't too much work, and if it fits into my other activities, and if I can get it in a week".

If being a successful powerlifter is not something that you *really want*, then it will never be something that you achieve.

If you are going to accomplish anything in *any* part of your life, you have to have a burning desire to get it. Nothing of consequence comes to people who operate the way Woody Allen describes when he says: "...90% of life is just showing up...." In real life, Woody did not get where he is by simply showing up. He is a hugely talented guy who had a burning desire to succeed and then worked his butt off, and still does every day at age 80..

If we assume you have a burning desire to be the best lifter you can be, then the next ingredient in success is _persistence._

Perhaps the best definition of the most important factor for success in the gym (or any other pursuit) is a quote from Calvin Coolidge quote from about 90 years ago:

> "Nothing in this world can take the place of persistence. Talent will not; nothing is more common than unsuccessful people with talent. Genius will not; unrewarded genius is almost a proverb. Education will not; the world is full of educated derelicts. Persistence and determination alone are omnipotent...."

Limiting Beliefs

Desire is a necessary driver of success. However, a lot of people are stopped dead in their tracks by their limiting beliefs about their own potential.

It is virtually impossible to overcome obstacles if deep down you *really believe you can't do what you want to do.* A lot of these beliefs are unconscious, or at least have never been brought to your attention.

We have all heard motivational gurus say to an audience "you can do anything". There are some real limits to what you can actually do, but far fewer than most people realize. The key is whether there are pre-defined limits on what can be achieved, or no limits.

Let me use an example of a situation where there are overwhelming pre-defined limits.

It is common for young men to dream of becoming professional basketball players. The problem is that there are only a miniscule number of positions available. The total number of NBA basketball players is only 384 (32 teams with 12 players). How many players are trying to fill these positions in any given year?

Assume that there are 12 players on each of the 330 Division I college basketball teams in the United States. That would make just short of 4000 college players in any one year. Add to that the 350,000 high school players in the US, and another 150,000 in Europe and the Americas. For the moment ignore the half million players in China.

Each year only 20-30 new players enter the NBA…from the pool of at least a half million. That means the fraction of new players who will actually get to suit up for an NBA team is about 1 in every 100,000.

Getting to the NBA means competing for something that has immensely restrictive pre-defined limits.

However, there are other highly satisfying pursuits where there are NO pre-defined limits. If you select a goal that has no pre-defined limit, eventual success will be determined by your desire, creativity, commitment, determination and hard work. When there is no fixed limit on accomplishing your goal, the odds for success become drastically better.

For example, if your aspiration is to become financially well off, about 5% of the US population have a net worth over $1 million. That is roughly 16.5 million people, with no limit on more people succeeding. Compare this opportunity with the fixed limit of only 384 positions available in the NBA.

That's why you need to focus your energy on activities where there is no _pre-defined_ _limit_ on accomplishment.

When you apply this principle to strength and fitness, you are not limited by anything but your own desire and willingness to work hard. But, there may be some lingering doubt in your mind about this.

The thoughts and assumptions you have in your mind about what is *really* possible for you can be your biggest obstacle to your own success. Self-limiting beliefs are ideas a person has that they accept as "true". In reality these beliefs are nothing more than mental images that have little to do with reality.

Let me introduce you to some of the most insightful research ever done on the issue of self-limitation.

Psychologist Carol Dwek did extensive research on how people see their opportunities to succeed. What she found was that most people had unexamined assumptions about their own potential that either limited or facilitated how much they could achieve.

These assumptions were largely unconscious. The most common assumption was that to achieve success in any given endeavor, a certain amount of "talent" was needed. This talent was defined as the "natural ability" or "gift" that people had for a given undertaking.

Most people believed that they did not have the "gift" or "natural ability" to do many things that they might desire to do. But because they *believed* that "natural ability" defined how far they could go, they accepted low achievement as the best they could hope for.

This is called the <u>*fixed mindset.*</u> In this view of the way the world works, your potential future is limited by the store of "talent" you were given at birth.

Many people believe that they don't have the "talent" to succeed at such diverse things as mathematics, music, sports, business, relationships, etc. The "talent=success" idea assumes that people who succeed at something do so *only* because they are "naturally gifted".

It follows that if you assume you are "untalented" in an area, you will accept very low achievement in that area as being "normal", or to be expected.

In dramatic contrast to this assumption is the idea that you can attain unimaginable success based on your own hard work, determination, cleverness, etc. There are some limits on potential achievement, but far fewer than would be imagined. This is called the <u>*growth mindset.*</u>

The growth mindset assumes that any person's potential is basically *unknowable* at the beginning of an undertaking. There *may* be limits, but there is no way of knowing in advance what these limits are.

What Dr. Dwek and her research team found was that simply making university students *aware* that they were making *assumptions* that limited their aspirations made a gigantic difference in how they saw their own potential in life.

If they assumed they were limited by their so called "talent", then they saw limited chances for success in many areas.

However, when confronted with the fact that this limiting assumption was *nothing more than a "belief" in their mind*, the students suddenly saw a whole range of options open up.

The students quickly embraced the idea that they could achieve many different things if they worked hard enough. This was a liberating notion rather than to simply accept the idea that they were chained down by a "lack of natural ability".

This was the real life validation of the quote above by Calvin Coolidge. Remember a key part of the quote:

> "...(talent alone means little), nothing is more common than unsuccessful men with talent...."

Once you have the burning desire to succeed <u>nothing</u> is more important than persistence and determination. There are some limits imposed by so called "talent", but these are so minor as to be almost irrelevant.

My message is don't ever start a new activity by assuming that you have limitations. How far you can progress in 99% of human activities can <u>*never be predicted in advance*</u>.

Never assume that you can't accomplish some astonishing things in powerlifting or almost anything else. The key will be how much you apply yourself to the task.

Throughout my career both as a lifter and as a scientist, I often had people say things to me like, "you're successful because you are so damn smart", or "you're good because you are a natural athlete".

Rubbish!

I may have been given some modest genetic gifts, but to assume that any achievement comes because of talents I was given at birth is completely discounts all the work I put in trying to become good. I spent thousands of hours working to achieve the things I accomplished. Along the way, I saw people who were perhaps more "naturally talented" than I and failed to accomplish anything.

Let me give you a couple concrete real world examples that will illustrate this point.

I used to train with a lifter who had almost unlimited potential. He acknowledged that he had great potential, but never accomplished anything. In part this happened because he never bothered to "train smart" and avoid injury. He always had the convenient excuse that he was "injured" and could not train hard. The prospect of trying hard and failing seemed to dominate how he thought about his potential. In short, it was better to have an excuse for never reaching his potential than to fall short if he actually tried.

On the other hand, I know a couple of lifters who have good, but not great, athletic ability. Each of these men accomplished some mind blowing feats. Each had a burning desire to be good, did what they needed to do to get better, and worked intelligently at their craft over time to the point where they became world class lifters.

What DO you <u>intend</u> to accomplish? – The power of intention

Let me begin by making a critical distinction that may seem trivial on first look. It is another aspect mindset that is often the difference between success and failure.

There is a huge difference between the power you have when you "want" something as opposed to defining the situation in terms of what you "intend" to accomplish.

When you "want" something, it means you have already defined yourself in terms of being in a deficit situation. This is something you "don't have" for whatever reason. When you define a goal in this manner, it already puts you in a weakened position.

When you set your goals in terms of what you "intend" to accomplish, you automatically become much more empowered. This is not just a semantic distinction; it is a statement that makes you *feel* differently about what you are doing. If you intend to do something, you assume that you have the power to accomplish it, and you are in the process of doing just that.

The power of intention is huge, and it should pervade everything you do as you pursue your goals.

For example, your long term goal may be to squat 500 pounds in competition. On a daily basis, your *intention* is to do the workout exactly as planned. You never put yourself in the position of "I hope I can do this". If something prevents you from realizing your daily intention, that will do nothing to divert you from your long term intention.

Let's look at another example of people "wanting" something and "hoping" they can achieve it.

Every January a zillion people join health clubs and start working out. Most "want to get in shape" or something like that. Unfortunately, I suspect that most of them don't believe it is possible for them (fixed mind set) and they simply "want" to get in better shape than they are now.

According to industry statistics, 90% of the new gym members quit within a month of signing up.

In my opinion, the 90% who quit never make the transition from "wanting" to be fit to *intending* to be fit. Instead, I think they probably see themselves as deficient or "not very fit". Instead of seeing themselves as being "on the way" to their objective, they see themselves as permanently lacking.

What about the 10% who stay on? What keeps them training while the other 90% have stopped?

Clearly I think that most have had some experience in the first month that helps them develop the notion that they *will* be successful. They have a dream about getting in shape and getting where they want to go. The ones who stay on have developed at least a strong *intention* to succeed if they didn't already have it when they started.

The point is that each of them has embraced some part of their experience in the first month. They see their training as something they *intend* to continue. Training is now part of what they *see themselves doing.*

Step 1: Know where you intend to go.

Earlier I quoted powerlifting great Andrew "Bull" Stewart, as saying:

> *"If you have no plan, your plan is to fail"*

Your plan begins with knowing *exactly* (not vaguely) where you intend to go. An exact statement might be "I intend to do a 500-pound squat in competition". A vague statement would be "I want to improve my squat". In powerlifting, just like any other human activity, knowing what you *intend* to accomplish *in very specific terms* is absolutely critical.

One of the most powerful tools at our disposal to make changes is *setting specific goals.*

A goal is something tangible that you have *chosen* to pursue. It is concrete, measurable, and has identifiable steps along the way from where you are now to where you want to be. Goals are great because they focus your energy on a future condition that you intend to achieve.

There is a well-known story about the power of goals that followed the graduating classes from Yale University over the course of their working careers. About twenty percent of the class had set goals for their careers when they graduated. The remaining eighty percent did not.

Researchers tracked the progress of each member of the graduating class for three decades. At the end of that time they found that the 20% of the class who had set goals had earned more money in their careers than the combined earnings of the remaining 80%. This is a dramatic example of how powerful goal setting can be.

First, a goal has to be specific and measurable. It distinguishes between plans and daydreams.

Daydreams are nothing more than a wish, unconnected to a plan or an implementation strategy.

Real goals are things that you can control. You alone are responsible for doing what is necessary to get from where you are now to where you intend to be. You control doing all the things needed to become the best you can be.

Step 2: Create a training plan

Goals alone are pretty useless unless they are linked to a *plan* for reaching them.

Here is your mantra: "*strength is a skill, and skills can be learned*"

In Chapter 4, I showed you how to create a training plan. This plan was to prepare you for doing your best possible lifts at pre-determined dates during the year. Executing the plan required working on learning many different skills so that you could continue to improve.

Your plan is your personal template for improving all the things necessary for you to become a better lifter.

Step 3: Motivation and Support

Once you have a dream, you need to have it nurtured and supported. This is critical, because when we try to do something alone, we can fail for many reasons.

Training partners can be very helpful for keeping you on course. They also help with other matters during the workout such as spotting, loading and assisting with equipment.

If a dependable and highly motivated training partner is not available, develop some community support, either by training with a group of other lifters, of joining an on-line group.

Training alone can be more difficult, but it should be no bar to your long term success. I spent most of my lifting career training alone as it was nearly impossible to synchronize my work and travel schedule with other people. But at times, I trained at a gym where there were there was a good coach and a group of first rate lifters.

Step 4: Commit to continuing improvement

Once you learn the basics of some skill set, improvement comes from carefully working on the details that are needed to achieve *mastery*.

I see most people ignore the need for focused work on critical details. They simply plow ahead doing a lot of "work" without getting any better.

If you want to *significantly upgrade* your lifting, you need to be focused on improving the *details* of your performance. It is always the little things that will be the difference between improving continually or stalling out at a level well below your actual potential.

Step 5: Implement the training plan – the Action step

All the planning in the world is useless unless the plans are converted to <u>*action.*</u> Getting down to the work of training and improvement is where all the payoff comes.

Implementation means that you begin using a systematic approach to practicing and perfecting all of the small changes needed to make continuing improvement. This is the Japanese principle of Kaizen.   Great improvements come from improving a large number of small things, each one making a tiny positive change.

In powerlifting, the principle means *continually* making incremental changes to your strength, small improvements in technique, and other abilities as a lifter. The net effect is continuing improvement over time.

Making Major Progress in Small Steps: The Principle of Kaizen

All humans find that making changes in the way they do things is difficult. In part this is because we evolved in the wild where our survival depended on staying "safe". Evolution did not reward early humans who took chances. Thus, we develop "habits" that are familiar and seem like they don't put us at risk.   It is hard for us to change something that seems to be working.

Clearly, we are hard wired to resist making changes that require us to leave our "Familiar Zone".   How then do we ever make any progress that requires us to do new things?

Making Small Changes: The principle of Kaizen for Powerlifting

There is a muddled belief held by many people that improvement in a sport or any other activity comes when they can find "that one big thing" that enables them to go from average to super. The idea that there is one single thing that can suddenly make a huge difference in performance is completely illusory. There is no "magic bullet".

There is no shortcut to succeeding as an athlete, a musician, mathematician, businessman, parent or anything else. Success in any endeavor comes from learning one small thing at a time. Persistence means you will learn from conscious practice, trial and error, and many other ways of working to constantly improve your skills. Eventually you will *master* your craft.

The only overnight successes are those that happen in fiction or fantasies.

Remember: "Strength is a skill and skills can be learned".   You *learn* how to become strong one *small* step at a time. Many small steps yield a giant improvement.

Every training session is an opportunity to become a little bit better at some aspect of your chosen endeavor. You are getting stronger bit by bit, and by small improvements in your skill as a lifter.

How successful is this strategy?

It is behind the massive success of such great companies as Toyota, Sony, and Toshiba. It is the backbone of the practice that built Japan, a nation the size of California with a population of only 120 million people, into the third largest economy in the world behind the US and China.

The principle of Kaizen is that improvement is a process that can be accomplished by constant attention to the details of performance. Big improvements come from wringing every possible advantage or efficiency from every part of the process. Each of these improvements may be small, but together they become huge.

As a lifter you have only two resources to spend: time and energy. When you waste either, you limit your chance to make progress. The best way to make the most of your valuable time and energy is to *seek improvement every time you train and in every possible place.*

Embrace the principles of Kaizen in your training and you will succeed far beyond what you imagined was possible.

Here are *eleven practices* that embody the notion of Kaizen as applied to powerlifting.

Why did I select 11 practices as opposed to 10 or 12? Perhaps because the Japanese have a preference for odd numbers, and after all, the number 11 is a prime number. Clear enough?

Practice #1 – Focus your training intentions for every workout.

For most lifters the "workout" begins at some ill-defined time when you have dressed, shot the breeze with some people in the gym, finished a few "warm ups" and are ready to do work sets.

In my view, the mental start of your training session should begin as soon as you get out of your car and begin walking into the gym. Before you even walk through the door of the gym, you should have mentally rehearsed what you plan to do during the training session.

As you walk into the gym, you're getting your mind ready to do exactly what you have planned to do in this training session. Your clear *intention* is to do what you have written in your plan.

Practice #2 – Proper workout clothing and equipment

When you select workout clothing, the entire focus should be on functionality. Does it help you do heavy training? Does it keep you warm (or cool)? Does it remove the sweat so that you can grip the bars properly? Does it feel good when you wear it?

Forget wearing t-shirts that announce how bad you are, or other "fashion statements". They are frivolous and are irrelevant to what you are doing.

You should always have the proper gear in your bag so that you never need to think about equipment issues during your workout. This includes such things as shoes, wraps, belt, chalk, shin guards, or any other equipment you use during a training session. Make sure it is in your bag before you leave for the gym so that it is always there when you need it.

Practice #3 – Be in complete control of your mental focus

I strongly suggest that you *never* wear ear buds or head phones during the time you are in the gym. They are a distraction and for some, a crutch.

If you think you need music to get you "jacked" for training, you have not trained your mind to *do* serious lifting. You should consciously focus on being able to get yourself mentally ready to put out full power without relying on any outside stimulus.

You never see martial artists relying on head phones to dial up their intensity. You need to adopt the same frame of mind. You must train yourself to have *total* control over your own focus and intensity.

I strongly suggest you leave your cell phone in your locker for the same reason. You should not allow *any distractions* during your workout.

I'll give you a strange but true personal example of what I mean.

When I was training for the Masters National Championships back in the 90's, the great Bull Stewart was coaching me. The gym was on the 12th floor of a 50 story office tower in downtown Seattle.

I was on the second rep of a set of five deadlifts when (for real) a serious earthquake struck. I finished the set while the earthquake was making the building rock and roll! When I put the weight down after rep five, both Bull and I hustled into a doorway and watched the building sway like we were on a ship at sea during a storm.

This may not have been the smartest thing I have ever done, since the roof tiles or a light fixture could have come down on my head. But, it illustrates the idea that you cannot allow distractions to divert your focus when you lift.

Practice #4 – Practice your warm ups.

Over 95% of everyone you see training in a gym will simply "flop and thrash" through a bunch of movements to get ready to lift. In contests I have seen people do endless sets of a lift to get "warmed up". This wastes energy, but more importantly it teaches your body to be very lazy and not quickly become mobilized for a big lift.

Adhere to the following rule:

Practice so that you can be ready for a heavy lift with the <u>absolute minimum</u> of warm up reps.

This idea came to me from the martial arts. In judo, karate and other martial arts, people trained so that they could be ready to go into a full fight with little or no preparation. It was once expressed to me that "you have to be ready to go if you just stepped out of the shower".

What this requires is that you engage your mind to tell your body that "we are going to lift big iron NOW". You then practice using as few warm ups as you can to be ready for a given lift.

When I was competing, I would routinely do a total of four reps to go from "cold" to being ready for my first attempt. In the squat, I would do *two* perfect reps at 135, then do perfect singles at 225, and 275 before my opening attempt at 325.

By contrast, I would see other lifters doing 5-10 reps with 135, then 3-5 with 225 and so forth. They would work their way up to their first attempt with anywhere from 15-25 individual reps done in "warm ups". This is a massive waste of energy.

To get to the place where you can be ready to do an opening attempt by doing no more than five total reps in warm ups, you need to *practice minimal warm ups every training session.*

When you're doing heavy squats, you literally practice the warm up you will use in a meet.

It may take you a few weeks to get comfortable with minimal warm ups, but it should be something that you begin working on immediately, and use it every training session. By doing it every training session, your body will automatically be ready to go "from 0 to 60" when you are in a meet.

Practice #5 – Practice Minimum set up movements

How many times have you seen a lifter doing a heavy squat take the weight, then take seven to ten individual steps to finally be in position to do the lift? I have seen this so many times it is mind boggling. Most lifters don't seem to recognize that the longer you have to hold the weight on your back, the more difficult it will be to do the lift. The weight gets heavier by the second.

Practice your set up for squat, bench press and deadlift so that you literally do it exactly the same way every time, and with the *absolute minimum* of effort and movement.

For example, in the squat you should practice being in perfect position to do your attempt *by taking no more than <u>three steps</u> out of the rack.* Your first step should get you back a few inches from the rack, and then the next two should get your feet in perfect position for your attempt. Some lifters can do this in two steps, but three allows you to insure perfect foot position.

I use the squat example to show how practicing a perfect set up can give you an advantage over your opponents who may be prone to take needless time setting up while supporting a heavy weight.

Setting up for the bench press should be just as efficient and involve a minimum expenditure of energy. I have actually seen a few dimwits fail to get into position to bench press within the 60 second time limit for starting the lift. Don't ever be that guy.

Practice #6 – Do perfect reps every time, regardless of the weight

Earlier I told you about the coach who taught his lifters to squat by letting the weight push them below parallel. This produced regular failures in part because few of the lifters had any idea what a good competition squat felt like. They were always "hunting" for proper depth.

If you want your brain to have one single program in it called "squat" then practice every rep to the same proper depth. Regardless of the weight you are using, you should go to proper depth and use the exact same form you would use if you were doing a competition lift.

One of my friends who is a phenomenal bench presser always used exactly the same technique whether he is pressing 135 or 635. He rarely misses a lift in competition.

Perfect technique is just as critical in all reps of the deadlift. If you slop around with a light weight, the chances are you will revert to poor form when things get heavy.

Practice #7 – Practice returning the weight to the starting position

In a contest, failing to wait for the referee's command to "rack it" has cost thousands of lifters some very hard earned attempts. Having spent 20+ years as a ref, I can assure you that almost every lifter (including me) has at one time or another completed a super lift, and then failed to wait for the "rack" command. The result is "no lift".

To drastically limit the possibility this type of error, you should practice waiting at the completion of every lift for the "rack" command. You can have a training partner call this out, (which is best) or pause for a second or two and say the command to yourself.

What this does is build a habit of waiting for the commands that you will hear in a meet. This becomes automatic and you never have to "think" about it. This practice will save you a lift (or more) on some occasion that can be the difference between major success or frustrating failure.

Practice 8 – Work on your balance and coordination

One of the things that will significantly impact the power you can put into your lifts is your balance and intermuscular coordination. You need to be conscious of focusing your attention on how you stand when lifting. If you don't have a solid stable base on your feet, then you will dissipate your effort and achieve sub-optimal results.

Working on balance is something that few lifters actually do. However, it will be one of those things that you can do that gives you an edge, perhaps a significant edge on your competitors.

The most basic skill you need to master is using the inside half of your foot (the big toe half) as the place from where you do your power pushing. The outside half of your foot is primarily for balance. Your 2nd and 3rd toes are the anchors for your stability.

Regularly practice insuring that your feet are firmly rooted in the floor and your calf's flexed when you squat or deadlift. They should be completely tight and your foundation should be completely stable. If you are wavering or off balance, you will not be able to put full power into a lift.

You should work on being able to stand on one foot for at least 30 seconds at any time.

Intermuscular coordination is the foundation of being able to move heavy weights. Always exercise with free weights, and do compound movements that involve multiple muscle groups.

Avoid training on machines. In the words of one of my highly accomplished lifting coach friends; "machines will suck the athleticism right out of you."

Machines stabilize the weight in ways that you need to train your body to do. Using machines in training will deprive you of the critical skill development of controlling the weight in space.

Practice #9 – Keep detailed written records of all your training

The thing that makes Kaizen work is keeping detailed information on what was done, and what were the results. Your training records will be the only way you have of determining what is working well, what is not working and where your problems are emerging.

It is also the case that if you keep a record of your lifting, you will pay much closer attention to your training than if you did not keep a written record. What you write down is what you unconsciously believe is *very* important.

Keeping useful records means scrupulously recording every weight, every set and every rep you do during every workout. You should also write down any thoughts you have about what you discovered in each training session. It is often very helpful to write these down as they occur to you during the workout.

Recording this information when it occurs is critical, because your memory can never keep all the detail needed. You will have thousands of entries in your workout record in any given month. Make your life simple, and record everything as it happens.

From this you can do your own evaluation of what is working for you and what needs to be changed.

You can use a simple composition notebook, or one of the many apps available to record workouts. Being an old timer, I tend to favor the notebook because it is simple to use, and can't get broken if someone drops a weight on it. The choice or record keeping technology is yours, just so long as you *keep* detailed records.

Practice #10 The Power of Coaching and Community

Even if your motivation and commitment are off the chart, you can always benefit from good coaching and from training with other powerlifters. Good coaches can be worth their weight in gold. The company of like-minded athletes can provide huge benefits in both support and coaching.

There are *very few* good powerlifting coaches. Unless you live in a good sized urban center, finding a coach can be difficult.

If you want to find a good coach, it will probably take some significant effort. Searching on the internet can at least give you some possibilities to interview. If you train at a gym where there are powerlifters who compete regularly, you should ask them for recommendations. In any case, you should be prepared to interview the prospective coach and find out if he can help you.

Good coaches have always been competitive lifters for a long time and have learned their craft from both practical experience of "being in the arena" and working with other lifters who compete regularly. I don't know of any exceptions to this rule.

The fact that someone has a personal trainer certification means nothing when it comes to knowing about powerlifting training. In my experience fewer than 1 in 100 personal trainers have any idea how to even do a proper squat, bench press or deadlift. Their training is to assist beginners and fitness trainees.

The elite personal trainers will usually be specialists in one type of sport, and be absolutely excellent for that. I once belonged to a club where the top personal trainers had specialties in such things as racquet sports, triathlon, competitive bodybuilding, football conditioning, and so forth. They were great at their specialties, but they would tell you that you don't hire a coach with a background in triathlon to try to teach powerlifting.

What is a coach going to give you that no one else can?

Excellent coaches have the ability to help you master the many small things that are needed to become an outstanding lifter. They see things that are invisible to the novice. Any bozo can show you the elementary things, or you can watch a You Tube video. The real value of an experienced coach is that he or she can help you correct the myriad of small subtle things that make the difference between excelling or under-achieving. This is the principle of Kaizen.

When you find someone you may want to have coach you, it is important that you interview them before committing to work with them. The interview is for you to determine whether this person is truly knowledgeable and has produced top notch lifters, or whether they are blowing smoke.

The first and most critical question is whether they competed themselves and, for how long. I have never encountered a good coach who had not spent a lot of time competing. In my opinion someone who claims to be a coach should have competed regularly for a minimum of five years.

A second critical question is what current lifters do they coach, and how are these lifters performing. A good coach should have at least five lifters training with them (usually more) and these lifters should be competing regularly (two or three times a year).

If he (or she) seems to have the requisite experience and is training a group of lifters, you should decide whether you want to work with this person. Their personality should mesh reasonably well with yours or you are going to have problems working together.

When you select a coach, in most cases you will be selecting a group of training partners. Most often groups of lifters train together under the coach's supervision. You should decide whether you have any deal breaker type issues with any of the training partners. If not, charge ahead.

I should note that if you train with a specific coach, there is no reason why you can't opt for a training session from another coach. Every good coach has unique strengths. You benefit from learning from many skilled teachers.

During my career I was coached by several people. Each had some unique things that they taught me. I benefitted greatly from working with all of them.

Practice #11 - The Power of Community: Training Partners and Groups

If there is one thing that will consistently help you keep improving, it is training with other like-minded people. When all of your training cohorts are focused on improving their game, it automatically elevates your energy, commitment, and sense of being involved in a rewarding experience.

You will probably develop a sense of camaraderie with lifters who train under the same coach. This sense of community can be a powerful motivator. You support each other, understand what each of you is trying to accomplish, and help coach each other during training. In short, your training partners can make heavy training seem downright pleasant.

FUN

They also need to reinforce the idea that you are all improving. A good group of training partners will constantly work to encourage each other and convince them that they are on the path to success. In short, a good group of training partners will always encourage you to do your best and maintain a realistic and positive attitude.

Having a positive "can do" attitude during your training is really important. People choose to become powerlifters because they want to do it. There is no money in the sport, it is strictly for the people who have a *burning desire* to compete for their own individual reasons. You have to work hard for even modest success. Becoming the best you can be takes a lot of energy. In this environment, someone who has a negative attitude can kill others' enthusiasm.

Negative people literally suck the energy out of those around them. You need your energy for lifting weights, not dealing with another person's dark view of the world. You should do whatever you can to avoid negative people. Not only in the gym, but in the rest of your life as well.

You may have one person with whom you do most of your workouts. It is really important that this person bring positive energy to your workout experience. The most critical thing is that they share your degree of commitment. They don't have to lift the same weights you do, but they need to help you maintain your drive, intensity and focus.

Some powerlifters work out with their spouse, friends, children or someone else from the gym. These people can be great training partners. They can also create distractions. Their minds may not be into serious training to the degree yours is. Their schedules may not match up with yours. If that is the case, you need to evaluate whether to train with them or not.

During my working career I found that I had to work out alone much of the time. I had extensive national and international business travel. Often I had to work out in gyms far from home. Because of that, at times I found that I had to be responsible for my own focus, intensity and motivation.

But, when training at home I had the regular support of a community of powerlifters, coaches, friends, and others who always gave me positive vibes. When I trained on the road, I felt the presence of these people who gave me so much inspiration, support, feedback, and motivation.

It's about more than you

In the bigger scheme of things, your commitment to become strong and healthy has a positive impact on almost everyone around you. Your family benefits from having you healthy, your kids see a great example of how to care themselves, your co-workers benefit from having a confident and healthy person in their midst. In short, your training touches a lot of people who see you every day.

The society at large benefits from your commitment to being healthy and strong. With medical care costs going through the stratosphere, your individual commitment to taking care of yourself eases the burden on everyone else!

According to Dr. Michael Roizen, MD of the world renowned Cleveland Clinic, 87% of the *total* health care cost in the United States is spent on managing chronic conditions such as diabetes, heart disease, and conditions that come about because of *poor lifestyle choices.* The total cost amounts to billions and billions of dollars' essentially *spent for nothing.* We are paying for our own gluttony and lack of common sense.

According to Dr. Roizen almost 75% of chronic illness can be *improved or cured* by changing only four aspects of our lifestyle: don't smoke, eat better, reduce daily stress, and <u>*exercise!!*</u>

By being a living example for other people, you can magnify the positive impact you have on the lives of others. They may be inspired to improve their own lives from seeing what you do.

So you see…in the big picture, your commitment to strength, health and happiness can have a much bigger impact than you may have ever imagined.

Chapter 13

Nutrition for Power

This could be a really short section of the book…because the basis of good nutrition for building strength and power is pretty simple. I know it seems there are more diet and nutrition books out there than stars in the sky. However, the core advice is much the same in all of them:

- Eat "good stuff"
- Don't eat "bad stuff"
- Don't eat too much

And there you have it….

I'll try to keep the guidelines simple, because those will work for 99% of you.

Let's begin with a basic assumption: to be a competitive lifter you have to maximize your muscular body composition and minimize the fat.

So far so good…since you will compete in weight classes, it stands to reason that you want to have as much muscle as possible for your body weight. That means the lean lifter will always have the advantage whether you are competing at 148 pounds, 198 pounds or 242 pounds.

Extra body fat is highly beneficial only if you are planning an extended stay in the Arctic (or Antarctic).

So, my advice to you is going to be directed at building a lean muscular body.

This sounds like the same advice everyone is offering. Whether you want to go for the "beach body", get "ripped" or just look good in your clothes, the guidance you get is some variation on the three bullets above.

Let me begin by saying that over the course of my 60+ year career in sports, I have tried a lot of different nutrition strategies. I believe that *all* of them work to some degree, and none of them work if you only buy the book but don't follow them.

I'll stick to what I believe will work for most people...including you and me.

As many of you know, there are a lot of "diet crazies" dwelling on the internet who will maintain that their particular approach to eating (and living) is the only valid one in the galaxy. Their zeal and total belief in their own version of "the truth" about eating would be right at home in the Spanish Inquisition.

While the antics of these self-proclaimed owners of "The Truth" can be amusing, don't anticipate much new information. While a few will have some off the wall advice, such as that you can develop a God like body living on a diet of "possum and ground nuts", most will offer variations on well-worn themes.

Eat "Good Stuff"

The central theme in all solid nutrition strategies (including mine) is: "Eat good stuff".

OK...what is the "good stuff".

#1 – Protein sources: That is meat, fish, chicken, beans, eggs

#2 – Vegetables – All veggies

#3 – Water

All of these items are critical if you want to build a powerful body

To build muscle, you need protein...period! It is your choice what to eat for protein sources. Most like meat, fish, eggs and chicken. If you are a vegetarian, you will get your protein from vegetable sources

Vegetables give you a wide variety of vitamins, minerals, and carbohydrates to fuel your bod. Forget the noise about certain veggies not being part of our ancient ancestor's diet.

Water is essential to all digestive and metabolic processes.

Keeping it simple: Eat roughly ½ gram of protein for each pound of your bodyweight. Eat all the vegetables you want. Drink at least 8 glasses of water per day if you are between 170-220 pounds of bodyweight. More if you are bigger, less if you are smaller.

Don't Eat "Bad Stuff"

If the good stuff is pretty simple, the list of bad stuff is much larger.

Here are some basic rules that you can follow:

#1 – Avoid processed foods – those that come in a can

#2 – Avoid manufactured foods – those that come in a bag, like corn chips

#3 – Avoid high sugar "fat bombs" – muffins, cakes, cookies

#4 – Avoid bread and other grain products –

#5 – Minimize dairy products – milk, ice cream, cheese

Having read this list, you may be convinced that if you follow my advice, life may not be worth living. Life without ice cream and donuts? No chocolate chip cookies? Maybe you are thinking "Crap!!!! This guy is a sadist!"

I'm not suggesting you adopt a diet plan suitable only for low-carb psychos or Paleo Jihadists. I am suggesting (strongly) that you take steps to eliminate a lot of the rubbish in the "normal" diet that packs pounds of lard on your gut and leaves you weak and over stimulated at the same time.

Your goal is to fuel your bod with good stuff, and build muscle. Not fuel your bod with things that leave you looking like a strange balloon and feeling like the morning after downing a quart of gin.

There used to be a saying that if you eat crap, you will feel like it. I would amend that to say if you eat crap, you will *look* like it and feel like it.

So…think about eating as much *fresh* food as you can. Frozen is OK…but canned, preserved and otherwise loaded with additives to prolong shelf life is not. Start making your choices from the produce and fresh meat areas of the supermarket…not from the cans and packages.

Minimize the amount of sugar you eat….as in cookies, muffins, pastries, bread, and cereal. "Stealth" sugar is everywhere, often masquerading as "health food". Learn to avoid these like the plague. These "fat bombs" are often hiding in plain sight.

Let me give you an example. The other day I went into a "new age" coffee shop for a quick afternoon brew. Most of the patrons were "enjoying a relationship" with their laptops while sipping the fair trade ground on site coffee. Right at the counter were an assortment of muffins, cookies, and cupcakes with enough sugar in them to alter the outcome of a Super Bowl. They were however "gluten free", "organic" and of course endorsed by the baker as "highly nutritious".

I won't kid you…all of the goodies in the case were yelling at me with sweet little voices saying: "eat me, eat me, eat me, eat me…etc". I had come for coffee…and despite the chorus of little voices, I stuck with drip coffee.

Coffee shops are one of the worst places in the galaxy to get food to begin your day. I love coffee, and drink a bunch of it, but the poor commuter who stops in for a coffee and "roll" will soon find he has another "roll" to contend with…the one on his gut.

Next time you consider having a "bran muffin" for breakfast, you might remember that you don't really need to put it in your mouth. You could just apply it directly to your ass.

Avoiding most grains is another thing I would recommend. In particular, limit your intake of bread, rolls, bagels, pastries, etc. A lot of people have a mild allergy to wheat. Only about 5% of the population is allergic to gluten.

Significantly limiting your intake of dairy products is another strategy I recommend. Note that I said "limit", not "eliminate".

The main problem with a lot of dairy products is that they are difficult to digest for many people. On the other hand, products like Greek Yogurt, Cottage Cheese and milk have a huge amount of protein.

What I suggest you do is to run a *completely personal* experiment by eliminating wheat and dairy products from your diet for a few weeks and see what happens. You may notice significant fat loss and you may feel better. On the other hand, you may not see much change. Each of us is a little different and you need to know how *your* body responds to different eating patterns.

If you notice significant changes in how you feel and/or look you have a powerful indication of what foods are not good for you.

Don't eat too much!

Like it or not, in the big picture, *calories do count* when trying to either lose fat or build muscle. Your goal will be to optimize your intake so that you get adequate amounts of good protein, fats and carbs. At the same time, you want to eliminate the fat bombs, stealth sugar and allergens.

When counting your calories, everything that goes in your mouth counts. Some people seem to believe that if no one sees them eat something it doesn't count. Not so fast....

Then there are the "eat all you want" type diets. They are very popular. Unfortunately, for them to work you have to assume all you want to eat is small portions of exotic vegetables. If you "eat all you want" of chocolate chip cookies, peanut butter pie, and deep fried okra, you better plan on buying new pants every month.

If you buy into the idea that "calories don't count", then I have some wonderful ocean view property in Kansas you might want to consider purchasing.

The critical point for you is making the calories (aka. "Food") you eat be the right stuff to help make you lean and strong. In modern America this can be tough since the food industry regards your mouth as a "business opportunity". Your digestive system is for the "transformation" of their products.

For example, consider the "food like items" you see for sale in mini-marts and other retail establishments. They are manufactured from edible materials (eg. Corn) and are certified by the Government to be non-lethal. Such items have been engineered to taste good, and give you an eating "experience" that will encourage you to chow down the entire bag in one sitting...and buy more.

Some of the most infamous food like items have the quality of being mildly addictive. Not that you are likely to commit an armed robbery to get tortilla chips, but these engineered foods are constructed so that you keep you buying (and downing) bag after bag.

Your basic defense is to use the muscle between your ears….and think hard about whether you want to eat something that gives you no real benefit…or even has a negative effect. Make a *conscious choice* whether to eat something, or not. If you go on autopilot, the chocolate chip cookies will win every time.

What do I do?

Probably the best overall approach you can follow is to begin by deciding what it is you *really intend*. I don't mean the usual frivolous "want" list like "be a millionaire" or "become a rock star". I mean what is it that you *really* intend to accomplish by doing power training.

Then, you make a *plan* to get there. **An unplanned life is <u>chaos!</u>** It means you do a lot of activity, but make little progress. An unplanned life means you are always responding to whatever is happening at the moment.

We all know people who are extremely "busy" who never seem to get anywhere. They never do anything but "fight fires" or respond to the crisis of the moment. This behavior pattern will make a person tired at the end of the day, but the chances of making any progress is zero.

I have often heard the comment that someone is "too busy" to do something…like exercise, or figure out what to eat so they can be healthy, or learn something new. What this amounts to is saying "I'm too busy to do anything important".

When you think of eating, an unplanned life means you are always at the mercy of immediate gratification. You are "hungry", so you get something to eat at the closest available source. Since you have no plan, there is no reason to expend energy seeking out good food over more quickly available junk food. Get the picture?

A plan makes you get concrete very quickly. Let's say you want to squat 400 pounds at a body weight of 175 within two years. You have to plan your training *and* your nutrition. That leads to a very specific set of things you will….and will NOT do.

On the nutrition side, it means that you adopt the attitude that you eat to build your strength and muscular endurance. You don't eat just to plug up the toilet. You make conscious choices about what foods are helping you reach your goal, and which are detracting from it.

This should lead to a mindset where your interest in crap edibles diminishes to the point where they will become almost irrelevant.

Here is a personal example: I obviously have a strong desire to be strong and healthy. When I shop at the grocery store I find that my attention is drawn exclusively to the fresh produce, fresh meat and fish, and to other choices that are healthy. The "chips and popcorn" aisle doesn't even register on my attention screen. I would have to think hard about where to find candy, cookies or cigarettes.

This is not an example of "will power". At one point I might have consciously denied myself certain food items, but after a very short time, I found that I wasn't even interested in a lot of the edibles that I used to eagerly munch without thinking about it.

The idea of using "will power" to deny things we "want" is a tricky concept. It leads to thinking that "I really want this (fill in the blank), but I can't have it". You can hang in there for a few days with this type of thinking, but eventually, the chocolate chip cookie will win. You really want it, but you are telling yourself over and over "I can't have it".

How does the cookie win? If you deny what you *want* long enough, eventually, you tell yourself "I *deserve this*" because (fill in the blank).

Denial of something you want, is a set up for failure. In the beginning of a new practice, you may need to avoid something, but you can't sustain your abstinence very long if all you focus on is what you want but can't have. There has to be a bigger objective that you *really* <u>intend</u> to achieve.

More to the point, you have to use your mind to understand that you have to eat and what you need to avoid. Develop a consistent strategy, and then <u>*implement this strategy.*</u> When you see the individual choices as *parts* of an overall strategy, you will find it is much easier to do them on a regular basis.

In short, each time you are confronted with a potential choice about what to eat or not eat, you won't have to make a decision. You *decided* only to eat the things that support your strategy, not treat each new situation as a "should I or shouldn't I" situation.

What's the Plan?

Begin with planning what you are going to eat each day for a week. Then go shopping to insure that you have the food you need on hand.

This is painfully obvious and very simple to say. Over the years I have been astonished by how few people actually put this into practice.

This format is exactly why the *Weight Watchers* franchise works. All the meals are pre-determined. No spur of the moment decisions, no agonizing over whether something should or should not be eaten, no fight with yourself over how big a portion to take. It is all planned out in advance.

This is no secret formula. But it run counter to our natural human tendency to respond to the immediate stimulus rather than defer gratification.

If you have been living without planning your meals, doing a week long plan the first time may feel like an exam in integral calculus. It may also feel like you are observing the rules of some obscure monastic order.

This is because planning what you will eat for a week is something you may never have done before. Like all new things, it is difficult to do the first time…and the second…and the third, etc. Think about how many tries' it took you to learn to ride a bike. Success did not come on the first, or third try.

Eventually, making and doing an optimal eating plan will be a *habit*. That is where you want to be.

Experiment on Yourself

As I noted earlier, there are literally thousands of diet plans available. But, for the most part people don't follow them. The problem is not shortage of information or viable alternatives.

In my view the problem that makes it difficult to impossible for a normal person to eat properly comes down to the following:

- Our normal human impulses are to seek immediate gratification. This is hard wired into our genes.
- Throughout history, human societies have had to deal with problems of food scarcity. Only in the past few decades have we been confronted with excessive abundance.

When humans evolved in pre-historic times, the ones who survived were those who ate whenever food was available. Since there was no guarantee that the next meal would be around when our ancient ancestor might want it, those who survived were those who ate something when it was available.

This pattern is clearly evident in the higher animals such as predator cats, monkeys and dogs. All of them have to hunt for food, and they consume it when they catch it.

One reason for this pattern is not gluttony. It is the fact that in the wild, food is *always* scarce. To survive, the animal must have a biological drive that keeps them constantly searching for food. All higher animals are *constantly hungry.*

As modern humans we have the same genetic make-up as our primitive ancestors. But, we live in the only time in human history *when food is abundant.* This abundance, or "over supply" of food only happened about 40 years ago.

Compared to the food available when I was a kid or teen ager, the amount and diversity is truly mind boggling. In the 1950's when I was growing up, the amount of food available in the super market was probably a quarter of what it is today. The choices available when dining out were few in number.

In the rest of the world mass starvation was still common. Famine persisted in India, China and other parts of the world until the 1970's. When the "green revolution" created vast new food resources, starvation on a mass scale disappeared.

What happened next was a rapid transition from shortage to plentiful to *abundance.* In the span of a couple decades, food production went from being a necessity to being an *expanding business opportunity.*

Because humans *enjoy* a variety of tastes and aromas, the food business went from providing basic "human fuel" to providing a vast array of products vying for a piece of the consumer's income. In short, food became a discretionary item, not strictly a *necessity*.

This is not because we "need" all these food choices for survival, it is because food items are designed to make the taste *very appealing.* When confronted with relatively inexpensive and appealing choices, consumers will buy. If they like what they bought, they will buy more.

There is nothing conspiratorial about this process of offering more choices to the consumer. We all like more and better choices in everything in our life space. This would include housing, clothing, transportation, computers, entertainment electronics and so forth. Food just happens to be one of the commodities where we have a massive number of attractive and inexpensive choices.

In the 1930's nutrition advice focused on "getting enough to eat". These days, diet and nutrition advice focuses on "eating the right things and not eating too much".

Which brings me to one of the main points of this section. Determining which nutrition strategy works best for you will require that you do some tests on yourself. This will involve trying certain diet/nutrition approaches for a few weeks at a time in your own personal experiment.

I'll begin by saying that for me the Paleo system works really well. Following this approach, I stay lean and strong.

You can test this approach out by simply eliminating all grains and dairy from your consumption. That will get you about 90-95% of the impact of Paleo. If you want to go completely Paleo, you will need to consult a detailed list of foods you should or should not consume. Check my website www.MidLifeHardBody.com for details.

You should also check out the Mediterranean Diet, and the Zone Diet to see if they work for you.

Remember, the best diet for you is the one that *you will stay on* and that *gets the results you want*. All of us are a little bit different, and what is good for one person may not work as well for another.

Another tactic worth trying

For people over age 50 it is important to remember that you don't need as much food each day as a teen ager or a kid in their 20's. Even if we stand up a lot during the day, most of us don't do heavy manual labor. So skipping some supposedly important "meals" may be something you want to try out.

There used to be an old axiom that "breakfast is the most important meal of the day". If you lived and worked on a farm or ranch, that was probably true. If you work at a computer screen, it may not be nearly as important.

Remember...each of us is a little different....

You might begin the day with black coffee (actually very good for most of us) and let it go at that until having a light snack in the early afternoon. Then have a solid meal at supper time.

What you are doing is a variation on "mini-fasting" where you consume all your daily calories in an eight-hour period, and then eat nothing during the other sixteen hours of the day.

You might try this out to see if it works for you. I say "try" because, you may find that you are dead when your training time comes around. You may also find that your body adapts to this regimen and you are able to train very hard.

Bottom Line

You need to find out what works best for you, and develop the plans and habits that keep you ready to do your best in the gym and in the other parts of your life. Nothing good will happen without a plan, and then executing and testing that plan. An unplanned life is chaos.

There are different approaches to eating and nutrition that will give you good results. You need to develop your own pattern and then stick with it.

Chapter 14

Overtraining and Injuries: Problems for the Serious Athlete

If you are going to become really strong and develop your capabilities to the max, you have to pay very close attention to the possibility of overtraining and sustaining injuries.

As you become more elite in strength sports (or any sport), you actually become more fragile in many respects than people who are unfit or cannot do half of what you can do. This is because peak performance almost always occurs right at the limit of your biological potential.

This is a hard concept to grasp for most people. The tendency is to think of extremely strong and fit people as being nearly bulletproof. The truth is somewhat different, and perhaps counterintuitive.

The most common problem for strength athletes (and runners) is that they don't manage the amount of training they do. The idea that "more is always better" seems to dominate the thinking of "gym rats". Let me discuss why this thinking can really be detrimental to your peak performance goals.

To begin with, you only have a certain amount of physical and mental energy to put into all parts your life on any given day. For people over age 50, the demands on this energy resource are considerably more diverse that for the typical 20-year-old. People at midlife (aka. "over 50) have to manage the demands of their jobs, family life, maintaining their home, their health, shopping, social life, possible volunteer work, and a lot of other things.

Physical training is one of many things that place demands on our limited supply of energy. Think of your total energy resource as having only so many units each day. You can use them however you want, but you only have so many.

We all know people who seem to have boundless energy and appear to do a huge number of things quite well. During my professional career I did a huge number of things every day (including working out) and had a family life, owned a small horse ranch, and had a social life. I also regularly traveled internationally on business, and if not traveling overseas, I was on an airplane to "somewhere" several times a month.

Over the course of my professional career I competed in foot racing and powerlifting, but obviously not at the same time.

Superman? Well....not quite.

One of the only reasons I could do this was that at a relatively early time, I discovered the way to work "smart" rather than just work "hard". I certainly can't claim I did this perfectly, or even adequately at times, but overall I allocated my energy pretty carefully and was able to get the most out of the gas I had in my tank.

Because of the professional schedule I had, it was really necessary for me to focus on the _quality_ of the training I did rather than simply the quantity.

Rather than developing a sound plan for achieving a goal, and then following it, many people will tend to overwork because they believe (wrongly) that they benefit from doing more and more work. *The truth is that once an athlete reaches a relatively high level of performance, it is far more important to work smart than it is to work hard.*

Beginners, novices and some under achievers tend to not do enough work to realize many (if any) results. In the case of people at the low end of performance, the root cause of poor performance is usually not doing enough work.

The same "more is better" logic does not always apply to athletes who have become advanced or elite performers. The basic reason is that the *elite performers are already doing a massive amount of work when compared to the novices*. For example, doing one full squat at your limit can take much more total energy than doing a complete "light" workout with weights.

The real challenge for elite performers is to identify what they need to do, and then do it with the limited resources they have in physical energy, recovery capacity, and mental focus.

Advanced and elite performers have already done thousands of hours of work to get to the point where they are. They have subjected their bodies to strains and stresses that novices could never imagine. In the process of getting to the top rung of their chosen pursuit, these individuals have developed their physical capacity right near the limit of their own biological potential.

As a consequence, the elite performers are at risk of crossing the line where their bodies can't take any more strain. When they cross the line, they get sick, or injured. That is why "training smart" needs to be the dominant theme for elite and advanced performers rather than "more is better".

Unfortunately, this situation is not widely recognized, and many lifters (like you) who want to excel wind up never coming close to their potential. Injuries and fatigue are the two main barriers to excellence once a lifter gets past the intermediate stage of training.

Training too much is like the proverbial "burning the candle at both ends". Doing excessive training burns up energy the same as excessive boozing and carousing.

When you work out too much (or party too much) a couple of the same things happen to diminish your overall energy reserve.

First of all, you are not getting the sleep you need to rebuild and recover. The biological consequence continually "running on adrenalin" is to over stress your adrenal glands and get into a condition called "adrenal fatigue".

In the early stage of this condition, you feel "tired but otherwise OK". If you keep pushing the envelope, you will experience what runners call "hitting the wall".

Despite all my good intentions, I have hit the wall on a couple of occasions when my enthusiasm got the better of my good sense. Let me tell you about them, since hopefully you will be able to avoid doing the same thing.

One of the most memorable came when I was preparing for a Masters National Powerlifting Championship meet. I forget what year it was, but it was in the late 1990's. The meet was a month away and I was getting into the home stretch of my peaking routine. I felt like I could lift the building where I was training.

Then came the workout where I abandoned "good sense" because it got in the way of my enthusiasm. By my standards, I was doing over the top in all three lifts. On heavy squat day my planned heavy sets went like they were warm ups. Why the hell not do more sets and do them with bigger weights?

My "reasoning" was that I was now one hell of a lot stronger than my peaking cycle had led me to believe, and it was time to revise my performance estimates upward.

I easily blasted through a few more sets of squats, much heavier than I had planned to do. Felt "OK" at the conclusion of the workout. I was covered in sweat and felt that I had really put in a solid training session.

The consequence of what I had done did not set in until my next workout. The warm up weights felt like they were 50 pounds heavier than they were. I never got close to what I had planned to do in the workout.

Again, my "reasoning" was that a good night's sleep would fix everything. Fat chance.

In the remaining time before the national meet, I never did get back to the level of strength I had when I decided to "do some more". I did "OK" in the nationals, but clearly had a degraded performance because I exhausted myself in a training session. Pretty smart, eh?

Now comes the part that is really important to you.

Remember, each day you only have so many energy "units" to do everything you need to do. If you spend more than you have for that day by working out excessively, *you are now in energy unit debt.*

When you are allocating a lot of your energy to training, you need to insure that you don't start running up a debt that can't be paid off (recovered) in one or two nights. It is possible to get so deeply in energy debt that you may take months to get back to an even balance.

If you are "in debt" and you continue to train hard, you will get in deeper and deeper energy debt.

This is just like running up a balance on your credit card that you have to pay off. If you don't over extend your spending, you pay things off every billing cycle. If the balance is too big, it takes a long time to pay it off and get back to even. If you keep adding to the deficit and don't keep pace with your payments, eventually you go bankrupt.

What kind of "energy" am I talking about?

This is basically the capacity of your body repair and restore tissues and hormones to optimal levels. This is not caloric energy, as in food.

Exercise breaks down tissues. When the body rebuilds them we have what is known as an "adaptive response". The tissues are re-built stronger than they were before. Over a period of time with focused training, lifters use the adaptive response of muscle tissue to create strong and high performing muscles.

The problem comes when we don't allow for the body to complete the adaptive response of rebuilding muscles and other organs. The body only has so many resources to repair and rebuild all the internal systems, including muscles and circulation system, that are used during a day.

When the total demand on the body for repair and restoration is exceeded by our activity level, that is when we get into what I'm calling "energy debt". All the restoration work is not completed before the next round of stresses hits. The net effect is for the debt to grow over time and never get back to the point where one or two nights' sleep will fully restore the bodily system.

Let me give you another example from my own experience.

At the times when I was training the most intensely, I would often get the flu or a cold. In one case, I was in nearly the best running shape of my life when I came down with a serious case of the flu.

What had happened was that by using all my bodily energy for training, I had depressed my immune system. I was susceptible to whatever bug was going around.

After I got wise to this, I have managed my energy expenditure so that it has been years since I have had the flu or any other seasonal illness.

There is a tendency for a lot of us to think that rules like energy balance don't apply to us. So often gym rats will believe that the cure for feeling like "dirt" is to "hit the gym" and get "some work in".

The only part of this that unequivocally valid is that breathing deeply expels a lot of toxic gasses from the body. The increase in blood flow is undoubtedly helpful is removing toxins through the liver.

Also, if your gym has a sauna, you can sweat out a grand array of toxic elements that will help your recovery.

However, if you are in an energy debt situation, adding more stress to your system by working out will give a temporary feeling of improvement, but will have added to your long term energy debt.

Over the decades I have been involved in weight training and sports, I have seen some careers and countless top performances thrown away by not training smart. This happens when athletes train past the point of diminishing returns, and the additional work begins having a negative impact on their performance.

For runners this often takes the form of running a bunch of "extra" miles in training, or doing too many interval sets. For lifters it has been doing too many sets with heavy weights, or just "doing some more work" because they feel good that day. These are called "junk" workouts.

The crux of "training smart" is to do your best to insure that you allocate your energy units in a way that lets you fully recover every 24-48 hours. This means getting the most out of the energy units you use in physical training. You have a lot of other important activities during your day, and it is essential that you have adequate energy to do them all.

In the programs in this book, I have endeavored to show you training programs that give you the "most bang for your energy buck".

Injuries

Physical injuries that happen in training often occur because the muscle, tendon or ligament that fails has been under stress for a long time and never fully recovered.

Over stressing muscles and connective tissue is constant issue with any athlete. Keeping away from injuries often means not "pushing" injured areas of your body when your good sense tells you that this is risky.

This completely goes against the culture of "no pain, no gain". The mantra there seems to encourage mindless charging ahead, regardless of any danger signals.

My slogan has always been "no pain, no *suffering*". Because as any athlete will tell you, there are two types of pain. The first is just the feeling that comes with hard exertion. That can be downright exhilarating. The second is pain associated with some significant malfunction in the body. That can be downright scary.

You want to avoid the second type at all costs.

The best guidance I can offer is to learn how to interpret the signals your body is sending you. If you are not used to a lot of physical activity, it may take a while to learn how to interpret these signals.

I'll assure you that pushing ahead with your training regardless of what your body is trying to tell you can be a recipe for disaster. I know several athletes who have shown far more guts than brains and suffered serious injuries in training as a result. In a training situation this is downright stupid!

Remember, the objective is to *win the competition*, NOT the workout.

For many of you the competition you want to win is "daily life". You work out to have a high quality of life. Having surgery and hobbling around with a ruptured tendon will not contribute much to a high quality of life.

What this means to you is straightforward. If you are injured, you can't train. If you can't train, you can't make progress. If you don't train smart, you get injured. If you over train, you dramatically increase your chances of injury, and almost insure that you will get sub-optimal results from the training you do.

Regardless of how careful we may be, training injuries do happen. When they do, it is in your best interest to immediately seek out the services of a good sports medicine clinic. Therapists who specialize in sports injuries know that you want to get well as fast as possible, and get back in the game. Other doctors may regard exercise as something akin to Medieval torture.

Chapter 15

Supplements and Performance Enhancing Drugs: A Cautionary Tale

Ever since I started lifting weights in 1955, I have seen a variety of products sold with the promise of "building muscle". Since then the "supplement" industry has exploded in ways that would never have been believable in the 1950's.

In the early days the main product was a protein supplement made from soy powder. Now most protein supplements are made from whey, but there are other products made with vegetables, eggs or soy. In short, lots of choices.

The type of supplements that are sold to weight lifters (and others) run the range from nutrition enhancements to hormonal products. Since the Soviet Bloc countries developed ways to make "chemically enhanced athletes" in the late 1960's, the number of performance enhancing substances has expanded exponentially.

The amount of "stuff" available that you can "take" is mind boggling. The summary advice I'm about to offer will hopefully help you make choices that will give you a really good quality of life. There are a lot of products out there that may give you a short term cosmetic benefit, and a long term life disaster.

As a person over age 50 the risks of using some compounds is really extreme. You should not take this risk lightly. Being aware and knowledgeable is really important to your quality of life.

Let's start with food supplements.

Food supplements: protein

Just about everyone who does weight training takes some protein supplement. There are a lot of protein powders for sale. Most are whey protein based. For the vast majority of lifters, these powders are completely adequate.

The rule of thumb for lifters protein consumption is that you should take one gram of protein for each 2 pounds of body weight (or 1 gram per kilo). If you are doing *very* heavy training, you can increase this to 1 gram per pound (or 2 grams per kilo).

There is an upper limit to how much protein you can actually absorb, (usually close to 1 gram per pound), so taking immense amounts of protein supplement will not give you proportional benefits. However, I have seen some of the dimmer bulbs in the gym taking vast amounts of protein with the hope that somehow they would quickly transform their stork like bodies into mountains of muscle.

The only thing that they managed to actually accomplish was to fill the toilet with very expensive "product", and significantly reduce the amount of money in their bank accounts.

Back to protein supplements. There are variations in the quality of different products that you should understand.

First of all, the mixing of some powders is not uniform, so while the label may promise so many grams of protein for each scoop, there may be a variation in the number of grams you actually get in a scoop. Sometimes you don't get anywhere near the promised amount.

A second more sinister situation is that some protein powders are "spiked" with other compounds that are not always displayed on the label. The purpose of the spiking is to introduce some banned compounds that will give extra cosmetic results. If the lifter believes that they got great results from the product, they will buy more of it.

There are some cases of "spiking" that are relatively well known in powerlifting circles. One involved a manufacturer who included anabolic steroids in every fifth can of their product. People taking the product got superior results (daahhh..). The product developed a loyal following until it was revealed that the company's marketing strategy had been to essentially dupe their customers into thinking they were getting great results from the protein powder alone.

In some other notable cases, professional athletes wound up failing drug tests (and getting suspended), because they had ingested banned substances that had been surreptitiously included in over the counter protein powders. Naturally, none of these banned substances was included on the label.

While "spiking" is (probably) no longer practiced, there are an array of protein supplements that are advertised as "super-anabolic" (blah, blah, blah, etc.). It is a good idea to avoid those products since they may well include banned substances that are not *illegal.*

I'll discuss banned substances in a later section, but for now you should know that the term "banned" does not mean "illegal". There are *some* banned substances that *are* illegal, such as anabolic steroids. But, there are a sizable number of banned substances that *are not* illegal (as in "legal") and are regularly sold over the counter in "health" food stores. For example, the product called DHEA.

The term "banned substance" refers to a performance enhancing drug compound that is banned from any athletic competition by the World Anti-Doping Agency (WADA). If a drug tested athlete takes a banned substance, they can be suspended from completion, as in the Olympic Games, major league baseball, drug free powerlifting and weightlifting, the NCAA, etc.

Back to protein supplements: My strong advice is to only take protein powders that are straight whey (or other type) protein and are not enhanced by many other compounds.

You will find many protein products with added free form amino acids, particularly L-Glutamine. This is perfectly OK.

You will also find protein powders and bars supplemented with vitamins and minerals. Again, this should be no problem.

One product that I recommend without hesitation is creatine. Daily supplementation with high quality creatine is something that is both safe, beneficial and totally legal.

Vitamins and minerals

Over many years I have tried taking many different vitamin and mineral supplements. I have read many many books and articles on the subject of supplements. In the end, I have come to the view that predominates in Chinese traditional medicine: don't take something unless you need it. When you no longer need it, stop taking it.

At one time I "pounded" vitamin and mineral supplements at a staggering rate. Without going into (embarrassing) detail, I'll tell you that at one time my monthly expense for vitamin and mineral supplements was about $160.

During that time, my diet was pretty good. But, I can't say that the massive amounts of pills made me feel any better, or gave my performance much of a boost.

While that was over the top, I'll retrace my steps to get where I am now, and what I advise you to do.

First of all, it is *essential* that you eat a diet rich in nutrients. Pills won't substitute for good food. You need to insure that you are eating lots of multi-colored vegetables, and fresh protein sources (meat, fish, chicken or vegetarian sources).

If you eat properly, the *need* for supplements diminishes pretty dramatically.

The vitamins and minerals in food are *bioavailable.* In other words, your body will actually recognize the vitamin compounds in food, and *able to use them!*

Very often the vitamin compounds in pills are synthesized in ways that make the vitamin molecule impossible for your body to absorb. The vitamin may be in the pill, but your body can't use it.

If you buy vitamins and minerals, you should purchase the kind that is called "whole food". This means that the vitamins in the pills come from actual food. As a result, they are highly bioavailable.

You should know that they won't be cheap. In vitamins and minerals, you generally get what you pay for.

One caveat. Every person is a little bit different. You may find that taking a few vitamins makes you feel much better than when you don't use them. On the other hand, if you believe you can't get along without a certain vitamin or mineral supplement, you need to run an experiment on yourself for about a week to see how you feel with and without the pill.

Now I realize that you and I are bombarded by "information" about various exotic potions that can work miracles if you take them. The hope is that you will believe claims like "a lifter in Oklahoma shed 100 pounds of fat, and put 200 pounds on his total by eating (our special product) essence of Nuthatch egg."

Most of these claims are the type of fertilizer you can't put on your garden.

If you are serious about becoming the best strength athlete you can be, you have to begin by insuring that you are eating the way you need to.

Having said that, I should make you aware of the fact that some supplements can actually be harmful to you.

For example, herbs are medicine just like pharmaceuticals. Traditional medicine used herbs to treat disease long before we had anti-biotics. Many of these substances are very powerful and can be dangerous.

While many herbs can be beneficial, be extremely careful about self-administering these compounds. At best they can help. Most of the time, you will not have a diagnosis that would justify taking something. Don't base your taking them on some advertising claim.

If you believe you want to use these compounds, I strongly suggest you seek out the advice of a naturopath or an herbalist. They are trained to advise you about the proper use of herbs.

There are also some chiropractors who are trained in herbal medicine. The bottom line is *don't* just take herbs because one of your gym buddies thinks he is getting "great results" from taking Cantonese Dickweed.

At worst, herbs can cause harm…just like other medicine. In some cases, catastrophic harm.

For example, I had a friend who was a top notch lifter and coach. He had been a fitness freak for over 30 years. He used an herb called yohimbe to help keep his body lean. Unfortunately, this herb also increases your blood pressure. My friend took yohimbe for years, until one day at age 55 he had a heart attack and died.

Was the herb the only cause of his heart attack? I have no idea. However, he lived a completely healthy lifestyle. His body was lean and athletic. He ate carefully, and neither smoked nor drank alcohol. He did not use recreational drugs. He had no symptoms of heart problems before the attack. He had no family history of heart problems.

But his blood pressure was "a little high" because of taking yohimbe.

Bottom line...taking herbs without getting professional advice is a risk I don't think is worth taking.

In regards to alternative medicine, I have educated friends who use traditional Chinese doctors as their primary care physicians. Because they live in Seattle, they have access to the large and renowned Institute of Chinese medicine. If you have access to this quality of care, you can probably trust the information and the supplements they provide.

However, if you live in a small town in Nebraska, it is unlikely that you will have access to a skilled Chinese herbalist.

Remember: only take a supplement when you need it, and stop taking it when you don't need it.

Anti-aging

There are few scams more widespread today than "anti-aging". Before going into a discussion of the rubbish being sold that make promises of eternal youth, let me remind you of a couple things you probably already know:

- Regular workouts with weights will help boost your testosterone levels significantly over time.
- Regular workouts with weights will increase your natural production of human growth hormone.

In short, your weight training can do more for you than anything to create great physical vitality and a good appearance. If you produce testosterone and human growth hormone from your own body, you will be in a "win-win" situation.

Now the other part of the story.

These days you encounter all sorts of "anti-aging" clinics and products everywhere. They are marketed aggressively because so many of our "Boomer" generation don't want to get old.

Using these products is very much like making a bargain with the Devil. You get to enjoy the benefits now, but pay a steep price later.

Consider the use of human growth hormone (HGH).

HGH is on the list of substances banned for athletic competition. Using it will get you tossed out of the Olympic games, major league baseball or any drug free amateur sport.

HGH is *not* illegal to use when prescribed by a physician. Remember the distinction between "banned" and "illegal". Plenty of banned substances are legal for over the counter sale and use by physicians.

There are thousands of people who take HGH regularly to slow the appearances of aging. How can it be bad?

First of all, it is really expensive. You will have to pay $500 or more each month to get HGH injections. For some of you, this is not anything to worry about. For others, it is a big outlay.

Now let's look at the dark side.

When you start taking a hormone replacement (injection), your body begins to shut down your own natural production of HGH. Over time, you become completely dependent on the injection for HGH. Restoring your own natural production of HGH at a relatively young age can be a long and painful process. At an advanced age, restoring your own natural production of HGH can be really arduous, if you can do it at all.

Here is some more fun stuff that happens by supplementing with HGH.

You see this "side effect" of using HGH in some bodybuilders, and it is something of a sick joke.

Extra HGH will cause many parts of your body to grow that you may not want to grow. For example, the bones in your head begin to grow. This often leaves the user with a caveman face look. If you crave the pre-human appearance, HGH is your thing.

Another quite unwanted "side effect" is that your intestines grow. This leads to the somewhat bizarre appearance I have seen in some bodybuilding contests where a man will have almost no fat (totally ripped) but have a pot belly.

If you like the pot belly look, HGH is your thing.

Most men I know would really like a flat stomach and a good looking face.

"Low T" and other phantom conditions

Another marketing blitz has centered on "Low-T", or (supposedly) reduced levels of testosterone. The idea being sold is that by taking supplements or prescription drugs, you can have the vitality of your late twenties when you are many decades older.

Most of this is marketing hype. Middle aged men may have lower testosterone levels than they did in their teens. However, for most this should make little difference in sexual capacity, or ability to build muscle. The hype comes in suggesting that by taking pills (or shots) you will get this huge boost.

The first question that any astute man should ask is "how widespread are clinically diagnosed cases of "low T"? The answer is that real "low T" is pretty rare. However, at times almost *everyone* feels the "symptoms" associated with "low T"; being tired, stressed, and run down.

Most people start taking testosterone replacements or supplements as an easy way to avoid finding the root cause of their (supposed) low hormone levels.

In most (not all) cases, low T levels come from lifestyle issues…. such as constant stress, not enough sleep, poor diet, and occasionally from too much exercise.

Too little sleep is the most common cause of feeling run down, having little sex drive and not being able to gain strength or muscle. Sleep is indeed the magic bullet for most issues around feeling run down. Unfortunately, most people want to ignore this because as a culture we are conditioned to believe we can take a pill and cure any problem we have.

Most of us have significant amounts of stress in their lives. Schedules, work pressures, money problems, family issues, relationship issues, etc. Constant long term stress from whatever sources will grind you down. It would be nice if you could take a pill and solve all these problems, but the problems are still there no matter how many pills get popped.

Too much exercise? Yah…a colleague and I did a research paper a while back that I turned into a short book called "Too Fit for Sex?". Basically, we reviewed the research literature on factors impacting T levels and found (no surprise) that middle aged men can significantly diminish their sex lives by putting too much of their energy into training.

How much is too much?

That will depend on the individual. Be aware that a lot of heavy working out, particularly on a regular basis, can cut into your sex life. Be prepared to experiment to find what works best for you by taking recovery breaks from training.

Like HGH, taking testosterone replacements comes at a price. Your body shuts down normal production of testosterone, and you become dependent on the pharmacy for both your muscles and your sex life.

There is a condition known as *hypo-gonadism* where the body does not produce enough testosterone naturally. According to the medical literature, this is a pretty rare condition. If someone has this, testosterone replacement therapy is needed. This condition is chronic and in many cases can never be corrected.

I have seen a couple professional athletes get drug exemptions for this condition and be allowed to use the cover story of "testosterone replacement therapy" to avoid being suspended. I'm smelling a big rat here….

Testosterone replacement therapy is marketed in many ways. For example, the practice of selling "bio-identical" hormones instead of "synthetic" hormones may sound reasonable. But, remember that whatever the source, taking hormone supplements will depress your body's natural production of testosterone.   That means you are not going to be able to quit the external supply without going through a prolonged withdrawal and adjustment.

Bottom line: "low T" is almost completely marketing hype designed to get you to buy something you probably don't need. The "something you buy" in this case is going to have very serious unanticipated consequences.

Performance Enhancing Drugs (PED's)

If you are a middle aged man (or woman) about the last thing you want to do is take any PED. There is nothing you are going to get from these substances that will be worth the price you will pay for the horror show that PED's will create in your body.

You should also be aware that using anabolic steroids or other substances banned by the World Anti-Doping Agency will get you suspended by drug free powerlifting associations. At 50+ you don't really want to deal with the embarrassment of being banned from competing in an amateur sport.

There is a huge literature on the impact of steroids and other PED's, and if you are inclined you can research it on line. I'll limit my comments to a personal note and a few observations.

The personal note is that in 60 years of competing in eight different organized sports (from high school to now), I have never taken any PED. At the tender age of 75 I have the body of a fit man at least 20 years younger...if not more. Not only am I fit and strong, I do not take ANY prescription medications. This is almost unheard of for someone of my age.

Anabolic steroids will give your lifting a boost. They do work to help you build muscle. No one ever contested that point.

One thing that is often overlooked is that if you use anabolic steroids, you have to keep using them if you want to keep the gains you made while on them. This is not a free pass where you make some dramatic improvement, then "go clean" and get to stay at the same level you were before. Remember, your body has lost the ability to produce these hormones on its own. You are dependent on the supplement.

It is also necessary to treat various medical conditions that emerge as a result of your supplement use. This means taking more prescription drugs to counter the "side-effects" of using anabolic steroids.

Overall, PED's are a high risk low payoff venture for anyone, and a really high risk venture for any man over 50.

Chapter 16

Entering a Powerlifting Meet: A Step by Step Guide

After you have been doing powerlifting training for a while you may decide you want to try competing in a sanctioned contest. Going from gym training to competing is a big jump, but one you will probably find quite rewarding.

There are a lot of things you need to do in order to compete in a real powerlifting meet. I'll walk you through them step by step. This will help you do your first meet with a minimum of surprises.

How a powerlifting contest is run and how you prepare for it

You need to know how a meet is run so that you can prepare for it. A lot of things will be very different than training in the gym, and the more you can prepare for them, the better chance you have of lifting well.

A powerlifting contest consists of three lifts: squat, bench press and deadlift done in that order. Lifters have three attempts in each of the lifts. The lifter is credited with their best successful attempt in each of the three lifts (in pounds or kilos lifted). The winner is determined by adding up the best lifts in the squat, bench press and deadlift to yield a "total". The highest total is the winner.

Each lifter will have three attempts to do each lift, for a total of nine attempts. Attempts in the squat are completed first, followed by the bench press and then the deadlift. To be credited with a successful attempt, each lift must be performed according to the rules and judged by three referees.

Before lifting begins, each lifter submits their first attempt (in pounds or kilos) for the squat, bench press and deadlift to the scorer's table on the official score card distributed prior to weigh in.

Individuals compete in groups of 10-15 lifters (called "flights"). Flights are typically made up of people in the same weight class, age group. In most meets there will be anywhere from two to four weight classes in a flight.

The order of lifting is determined by the weights selected by the lifters. The lightest attempt is first and the heaviest is last.

Every lifter in the flight will do their first attempt. The actual weight on the lifting bar will be changed as needed between each attempt. When the heaviest first attempt has been completed, the weight on the bar will be lowered to the point where the lightest second attempt will be made. Then all the lifters in the flight will do their second attempts. The same procedure will be followed for third attempts.

Following each attempt, lifters have one minute to submit their next attempt to the scorer's table.

Each lifter does their attempts in each lift in front of three referees. One referee will be in front of the lifter and the two others on each side. They will judge the technical performance of each attempt. A minimum of two of the three judges must believe an attempt was done according to the rules for the lifter to be credited with a successful attempt. If two referees or all three believe the attempt did not conform to the rules, the lifter gets no credit for the lift.

It is necessary for a lifter to get at least one successful attempt in each lift in order to establish a "total". If a lifter fails to get one lift passed in either the squat, bench press or deadlift, they will be out of the contest. This is called "bombing out".

The winner of the contest in each weight and age category is determined by the total number of pounds lifted. To arrive at the "total" the scorer adds up each lifters best performance in each lift. That is, the best lift in the squat is added to the best bench press and then the deadlift.

Now that you know the basic meet format, you can prepare to do a competition. The first thing to do is find a competition in your area.

Finding a meet

I suggest that you find out which powerlifting federations are active in your area. This is easily done with a Google search.

Where things get a little harder is deciding which federation you want to compete in. Here the choice is basically between drug free and not drug free.

As you have probably gathered by now, I have spent my entire career lifting drug free. I am a strong advocate of competing in this manner. For this reason, I recommend that you compete in either USA Powerlifting (USAPL) or AAU Powerlifting (AAU).

You can find a meet in your area that is sponsored by one of these organizations by going to their web sites.

In the United States there are a dizzying number of lifting associations. As I recall, the last time I checked a year or two ago there were over 30. Most are tiny with less than 100 members. One is very large, the World Association of Bench Press and Deadlifters (WABDL). This organization does not do full powerlifting meets as they don't include the squat in their events.

Outside the United States there is usually only one powerlifting federation in each country.

The reason that there are so many federations in the US has to do with the business opportunity of running a powerlifting federation. Each federation, no matter how tiny, will hold their own "national championship" and "world championship" events. This gives participants the opportunity to boast about "being a world champion", even though they might not be able to actually beat most local champions in a big association.

If you think this is odd, I agree with you.

The only US powerlifting association that has formal international recognition is USA Powerlifting. They are a member of the International Powerlifting Federation which is the organization that puts on world championship meets that are recognized by national sports federations around the world.

You should be aware of this before you sign up for a meet.

If all you want to do is be involved at the local level, your main choice will be between the drug free and drug permitted associations. If you develop a desire to compete on a bigger stage, then you need to be aware of the place each association may have in the bigger picture.

Once you have selected a meet and an association, you need to join that association. All of them require membership in the organization in order to lift in their meets. The annual dues may run between $25 and $50. You can usually register on line at the organizations web site.

Now you have to pay to enter the meet. Virtually every meet has an entry form on line that you can download and send to the meet director. The entry fee will vary depending on the expenses involved in putting on the event. If you plan for $80-$100 that should be about right.

Make a commitment to yourself and to the meet. Send your entry form in a month before the meet, not the last few days before the entry deadline.

There is always an entry deadline, typically about ten days before the meet. After that deadline, no new entries are accepted. This is because the meet director has to organize the lifting order, arrange for weigh ins, and order awards for participants.

My business partner and I put on three meets a year for a decade. Our largest meet ran for two days every year and had over 150 lifters. The logistics involved were mind blowing to someone who had never seen all the work involved in putting on a meet.

Commit to doing the meet early, prepare yourself and then be ready to do your best lifting. Don't be a wimp and wait until the last minute to enter.

Preparing for a meet: some early decisions

In order to do a peaking routine, I suggest you select a meet that is scheduled at least two months in the future. If your time horizon is shorter, do a shortened version of the peaking routine to get ready.

You will be competing in age groups and weight classes. You should find out what the weight classes are for the association running the event. Here are the current weight classes used by the USAPL and the older weight classes used by many other associations:

The age groups vary by federation, but in general all of them regard age 40 as the beginning of the masters age group. Some will have five-year age increments; others will have ten years. Check the rule book of your federation to see what they use.

USA Powerlifting and International Powerlifting Federation weight classes

Men		**Women**	
Pounds	Kilos	Pounds	Kilos
116.75	53	94.75	43
130.0	59	103.5	47
145.5	66	114.5	52
163	74	125.5	57
182.75	83	138.75	63
205.0	93	158.5	72
231.25	105	185.0	84
264.5	120	185+	over 84
264.5+	over 120		

Weight classes used by other federations and in use by all federations prior to 2010

Men		**Women**	
Pounds	Kilos	Pounds	Kilos
114.5	52	97.0	44
123.5	56	105.75	48
132.25	60	114.5	52
148.75	67.5	123.5	56
165.25	75	132.25	60
181.75	82.5	148.75	67.5
198.25	90	165.25	75
220.25	100	181.75	82.5
242.5	110	198.25	90
275.5	125	over 198	over 90Kg
Over 275,5	over 125		

You will compete in one of these weight classes. You can weigh up to the weight limit. There is no fudge factor here. If you weigh a tenth of a kilo over, you are in the next weight class up.

So, your next decision will be to decide what weight class you will enter. In general, you should minimize the amount of weight you have to lose in the month before the meet as it will cut into your strength.

Over the long term, it is to your benefit to be as lean as possible. Extra body fat does not give you any strength advantage. Your strategy should be to slim down *gradually* because when you do a "crash" type diet, you lose substantial amounts of muscle along with fat. Drop weight slowly and you will maintain muscle and burn more fat.

Your next decision will be whether to compete "raw" or with support gear.

Unless you have been training with support gear, you will be competing raw. This means the only supporting gear you can use are wrist wraps, knee sleeves and a lifting belt.

The USAPL has full competition in raw lifting. In fact, in most USAPL meets the number of raw lifters is usually double the number lifting with support gear.

Once USAPL changed their rules to promote raw lifting (2008), I noticed that the number of lifters going raw went from a few to almost 80% of the competitors.

You should be certain that the meet you want to enter will (or will not) have raw lifting competition. Using support gear adds a huge amount to a lifters total, thus putting raw lifters at a huge disadvantage if you compete against lifters using support gear.

Once you have decided what weight class to enter, and whether you will compete raw or equipped, you need to insure you have the proper equipment to participate.

Every lifting association has rules about what you *have* to wear when doing your lifts. All of them require a form fitting lifting suit. To my knowledge, *none* of them allow lifting in gym shorts, sweatshirts or any lose fitting garment. This is so that the referees can see whether you do the lift according to the rules. Specifically, none of your lifting performance can be obscured by lose fitting clothes.

The one piece lifting suit is required by all federations. This is exactly the same as a wrestling suit worn by amateur wrestlers.

For raw lifters, you should go on line and buy a wrestling singlet. You can find these at wrestling equipment suppliers. I recommend you get good spandex singlet as it will last you for many years. Pick out a color and design you like. There are few limitations on this.

Check the rules of your lifting association to see what their requirements are for footwear, sox, belts and non-supportive knee sleeves. You can only use equipment that is approved by the lifting association. The fact that your gym buddies may say it is OK means nothing if it is not on the official list of approved gear for the association.

Virtually all lifting associations require that tall sox be worn for the deadlift. The sox must come up to just below the knee. This keeps blood from getting on the lifting bar. The best sox widely available are soccer sox sold in sporting goods stores just about everywhere.

If you have questions about where to get approved lifting equipment, check out my web site at www.MidLifeHardBody.com.

A few words about cutting weight

One of the realities of competing in a sport divided into weight classes is that you have to do a formal weigh-in before you can compete. This is one of those reminders that this competition is very different from lifting in the gym.

Your first decision will be what weight class to compete in. I would recommend that for your first meet, you not compete in a class where you will have to cut any weight to get there. In your first meet, your goal is to establish a contest total. That will be demanding enough so that you should not add to your difficulty by having to cut weight.

My general advice is that if you have to diet down to the weight class, try to get to competition weight (on a real scale) at least a week before the event. If you ask me if I always did this during my competition career, the answer would of course be "no". So, I had experience with getting down to weight in the last few hours before the weigh in.

For the last decade of my lifting career, I had to weigh in two hours prior to the start of competition. That is the most demanding weigh in requirement of any lifting or amateur sports association. However, it is "real" in that you will be competing against people who actually weighed at or under the limit within two hours of the meet.

On rare occasions, I was in a meet where weighing in the evening before was permitted. This is pretty easy. There are even a few associations where you weigh in 24 hours before you lift, or longer.

The key thing is that all the lifters in your class will have met the same standard, whatever it may be.

Let's say you are just starting your peaking routine eight weeks from the meet. You are ten pounds heavier than the weight limit where you want to compete. Eating a strict Paleo diet should get you to the limit with no trouble. If you have two months to make weight, you can be in killer condition and make the limit with little trouble.

In order not to lose strength, try to keep your weight loss to 2 pounds a week or less.

If you do what a lot of us have done and try to cut down the last few days, then you have a different issue to deal with.

I had an advantage of learning how to cut weight in a hurry. In high school I was a wrestler, and an Olympic style lifter in college. Both were competed in weight classes, so I learned early how to use the sauna and some other tricks to cut down in the hours before an event.

When I started powerlifting again at the tender age of 48, I found all my old tricks still worked. But, there are some nuances that I believe are worth mentioning.

First of all, you need to *practice* cutting weight so that you know how different strategies work for you. If your first trip to the sauna is just before a lifting meet, you could be in for a nasty surprise.

The first thing you should find out is how much weight you lose overnight while you are sleeping. Weigh before you go to bed, and then immediately on getting up. This information will tell you how much weight you will lose normally while you sleep.

As a general recommendation, you should not try to cut a serious amount of weight. If you don't make it into the weight class you registered for, you are automatically entered into the next higher weight class.

But, if you are determined to make the weight limit I would *recommend* that you not try to cut more than 5 pounds if your normal weight is below 200 or 10 pounds if you normally weigh 225 or more.

The day before the meet, you can take an over the counter diuretic to help you eliminate extra weight in your colon. Usually this will be a pound or two depending on your body size.

Let's say the day before the meet, you need to cut from 187 to 183 pounds. Assume the weigh in is at noon, and you are at 187 at 7 AM.

First of all, you are not going to drink any liquid between that time and the weigh in. Normal evaporation through the skin means you will lose as much as a pound.

Going "dry" for a few hours is hardly an ordeal like having bypass surgery. You should rejoice if your opponents are losing their minds because of the pure torture of having to go without a drink for five hours. You won't think twice about this, because you are tough.

Go into the sauna about four hours before the weigh in. Stay in long enough to get a good sweat going. This will normally be in the 10-15-minute range. Don't decide to cook yourself or stay in the sauna so long you are really uncomfortable. Get sweaty and keep it rolling.

Be certain to wipe the sweat off. That will prevent it being re-absorbed by your skin. After your first session in the sauna, check how much weight you have lost on a reliable scale. You are focusing on how much you have lost in your quest to drop 4 pounds.

In all likelihood, you will have to make a few trips back into the sauna. Because you want to minimize the time it takes to start sweating, dress warm between each of your visits to the cooking box.

When you have dropped the 4 pounds you wanted to lose, you should go check your weight on the official scale being used for the meet. Remember, no other scale reading means anything. The only weight reading that counts is on the one on the *official* scale.

Assume that you are ¼ of a pound under the weight limit. You are "in". Now it is time to relax until the weigh in.

If you are ¼ of a pound over the limit, you have more weight to lose. You have to be at or under the limit...*precisely!*

Let me tell you about big mistake I made when making weight for a meet. I got down to the limit, and then *took a shower.* I wondered why when I jumped on the meet scale I was suddenly two pounds heavier than I had been three hours before.

When you are dehydrated (sauna) your skin will soak up water like a sponge. I had dried out than very deliberately soaked myself in the shower...voila...I quickly recovered the two pounds I had lost.

Check your weight at least 2 hours before weigh-in so that you know exactly where you are. If you have more to lose, back to the sauna. If not, lounge around in warm clothing.

Now, if you go to a meet that has no sauna remotely close by, you can utilize the delightful plastic "sauna suit" sold on line and in sporting goods stores for losing (water) weight. Put this baby on and with a little exercise, in a short time you will cook like a turkey in the oven. You will probably have to walk or ride a stationary bike.

Try not to burn up too much energy, but exert just enough to get sweaty and keep it that way.

There is another approach to dropping water weight that I have tried, but not used on a regular basis. This is the practice of super-saturating yourself up to 12 hours before weigh in, and then drinking nothing. Your body responds by urinating every possible drop and the reflex of shedding water continues right past the weight where you began. The net effect is that you drop several pounds by the body over reacting to being excessively hydrated by over urinating.

I have two reservations about using this approach to losing water weight. The first is that you lack any real control over how much you are going to lose. If you urinate like mad up to an hour before the weigh-in and you are still over the limit, what do you do? If you are using the sauna, you can at least get back in the sauna and drop another pound or two.

The second reservation is more serious, because it involves the risks of over saturation. Although this is a vanishingly rare scenario, I recall that during my running days a story came out about two runners who killed themselves by drinking too much water. They did this during a marathon. Excess water can dilute your electrolytes that allow the brain to send signals to your organs such as the heart. When this happens, no nerve signals reach the heart, and the person drops dead.

Granted, this is a highly unlikely scenario, but still one that gives me cause to be reluctant about over hydrating. I know how to deal with *de*-hydration, but not over hydration.

Bottom line on losing weight at the last minute. You should *practice* doing this so that your body is not shocked by the process, and you know how to control how much you lose.

By far the best practice is to lose whatever weight you need to through proper diet. This way you are within the weight class when you step on the scale just after you get out of bed in the morning.

But...let's return to your preparations for the meet.

Two weeks before the meet

With two weeks to go before the meet, you need to check your bodyweight to insure that you are where you need to be to "make weight" for the event. This is one of those signals that the event is a serious competition, not just a week-end training session with your pals.

Check your equipment to see if you need to purchase any new equipment, and take steps to get it if you are short.

You will be doing the last heavy lifts in your peaking cycle, because in the week before the meet you want to be resting.

If you want to be certain your entry form got to the meet director, give him (or her) a call and verify that you are entered. You can also ask any questions about the meet that may be on your mind.

If you are going to travel to the meet, you should insure that you have a hotel reservation at or near the lifting site. Very often the meet will have an arrangement with a hotel. Big meets will often be held in hotel ballrooms.

Meet week

You will want to do your last heavy lifting six or seven days before the event. If the meet is on Saturday, the last heavy lifts you should do are on the Monday before. Ideally, you would have done your last heavy lifts on the Saturday before the meet.

During the week your main focus will be insuring you are going to make weight, and resting.

Powerlifting guru Louie Simmons is reputed to have said "there is *nothing* you can do to get stronger the week before the meet...but there is a LOT you can do to *get weaker*...."

The things that will make you weaker are lifting *any* heavy weights. Even doing a moderate workout is going to detract from your meet performance. The best thing you can do in the days before a meet is rest. More sleep will do you more good than anything you can do in the gym.

You should check your equipment to make certain you have everything you need. Also, buy energy drinks, snacks or fruit that you may want to eat during the meet.

Pack your lifting gear in one bag, and insure you have the provisions you want available.

If you are flying to a meet, *take all of your equipment as carry-on luggage.* Never pack your lifting gear in luggage you will check at the airport. If you arrive at the meet site without a change of clothing, that is easy to replace almost anywhere. If you arrive without your lifting gear, you are screwed!

On the Wednesday before the meet you should know the schedule for the meet. That means the time during the day when you will lift.

These days most meets are divided into "flights". That is a group of 10-15 lifters (15 max) who will begin lifting at a certain time (with squats) and complete all three of their lifts before another group of lifters begins to compete.

This system was introduced in the early 1990's when the old format of lifting meets (clearly invented by the Devil) was killing the sport because it was so "unfriendly" to the competitors. In the (not so good) old days, the meet would begin with squats, and everyone in the event would finish their squats before moving on to the bench press. Once all bench presses were done, everyone would do their deadlifts.

My most memorable experience with this format came in a big regional meet in 1988 when I weighed in at 7:20 AM, did my first squat at 2:30PM, my first bench press at 7:45PM and my last deadlift at 1:30 AM. Clearly, the format from Hell.

These days one flight will complete their attempts before another group starts lifting. Usually one flight completes their squats, then another flight begins their squats. While the second flight is doing squats, the first flight warms up for the bench press. This means that any given lifter is usually done with all three lifts in 2 to 3 hours.

The entry form will include a preliminary schedule which is the meet directors *plan* for when different groups will lift. The final schedule will depend on how many people in each category actually enter the meet.

The final schedule can't be made until all entries are in. At that point, the meet director will organize the actual flights that will define when a lifter will compete. The final schedule will usually be *similar* to the planned schedule, but there are no guarantees. Everything in the schedule depends on who sends in their money and joins the meet.

A day or so before the meet, the final schedule should be available. This will tell you not only when you are scheduled to lift, but when you will weigh in. It is a good idea to check with the meet director to see when you will be lifting.

Rules on weigh ins differ from one association to another. The international standard for sports involving weight classes is two hours prior to competing. USA Powerlifting rules require that you weigh in 2 hours before you are scheduled to lift.

Other associations have more liberal rules. Some permit weighing in the day before the event. This means you might weigh in at 181 pounds and be about 195 by the time you walk on the platform to compete. But, as long as the rules are consistent, everyone is dealing with the same situation.

Some minor associations allow weighing in *two days* prior to the event. All I can say is "you can't be serious". Weighing in two days early makes a joke of competing in weight classes.

Night before the meet

Unless you live within a short driving distance of the meet, you will probably be spending the night before the meet in a hotel.

You should insure that your weight is where it should be for your weigh in. At most meets the weigh in will take place beginning at 7 AM. If there is a morning and afternoon session in the meet, the afternoon weigh in will usually take place around noon.

You should go through your equipment and general provisions that you want to have at the meet site. If you need to go buy snacks and sports drink, do it early.

Never do anything that takes energy. You can do all the celebration you want after the meet. Get a good sleep and be at the weigh in a little early.

If this is your first meet, you may be a little nervous. So are a lot of the other competitors. Being a little nervous before the start of an event is just one of those signs that this is a serious competition, not just another workout.

Day of the Meet

When you arrive at the meet check in several things will happen in fairly quick succession. First, you will have your lifting federation membership verified (or purchase a membership on site). Next you will be given your meet registration card. You will carry this through the check in process, and give it to the meet scorer's table when you complete check in.

Usually at this point, a meet official will check your lifting equipment to insure that it complies with the rules of the federation sanctioning the meet. If all your gear is OK, this will be noted on your registration card.

You should know the rules on what equipment is allowed and which equipment is required to compete in the meet. All of this will be in the federation rule book which is available on line. If you walk onto the platform for a lift attempt in illegal gear, you will not be allowed to lift. There is no fudge factor here. Know in advance what is legal and what is required.

Remember that one article of clothing that is required by most lifting federations are tall sox that come to just below the knees. These are required for deadlifting to prevent blood from getting on the bar. You should invest in a couple pairs of soccer sox which meet this requirement very well.

Next comes weigh in. You will be weighed by a meet official on a certified scale that is accurate to 1/10 of a pound. The scale will have been tested within the previous few months. In big meets it will have been tested the week before the event.

If you have been tracking your weight on a bathroom scale, a word of caution. Your bathroom scale is probably a piece of junk. If you have the chance, you should test your scale against one that has been calibrated for competition. This way you will be able to interpret the reading you get on your personal scale with an official scale that will be used at the meet.

The current crop of digital scales sold for weight management programs are usually pure crap in that they give you nice looking displays, but are rarely consistent and often wildly inaccurate. If you are going to buy a scale, search for one that is high quality, and then check it against a scale that has been calibrated for athletic competition.

The way you know a scale has been certified as accurate for athletic competition is that it will have a sticker pasted to the scale that tells the date of the calibration test, and certifying that the scale is accurate. You can usually find these at high schools with a wrestling program as they are required to be certified at least once a year. Some gyms will take the trouble to get their scales tested on a regular basis. But, you have to look for the certification sticker to know for certain.

But...back to the weigh in at your meet.

Weigh ins usually are done with the lifter naked. Some events will weigh you in underwear. Because of this, the weigh in is done in a private area.

The meet official will record your official weight on your registration card. If you are within the weight limit for the class you entered, you are good to go. If you are a pound or two over the limit, you will have a certain time, usually an hour or two, to either get to the weight limit or be entered in the next higher weight class.

You don't want to be in the position of having to lose weight in the last hour of the weigh in. Naturally, I have some horror stories to tell about this, but will spare you the pain. The best plan is to arrive at or below the weight and not have to devote energy to making weight.

Once you have a successful weigh in behind you, it is time to enter your opening attempts in the squat, bench press and deadlift. These will be written on your registration card *in pencil*.

Now, my advice on the weights you select for opening attempts.

Squat: My general advice is to pick a weight for your opening attempt that is equivalent to your *final warm up.* I would always recommend that you be very conservative on your opening attempt in the squat. This is the lift where you will be the most nervous, and have to establish your presence in the meet. If you make you opener, you are in the meet, your tension will dissipate and you can get more aggressive on your next attempt.

If you miss your opener in the squat, you will feel a lot of stress that has to be managed. You will typically do the same weight again. Once you have selected a weight for your opening attempt, you cannot lower it. For this reason, I suggest you select a very light weight for your opener.

My advice, select a very easy opener and make certain you are successful.

Bench Press – Your opening attempt on the bench press should be a weight that you can make relatively easily with complete confidence. You have no sense yet of how quickly you will get the "press" command, so you want to pick a weight you can do even if the head referee decides to go out for coffee while the weight is sitting on your chest.

Deadlift – Since the deadlift is technically the easiest lift of the three, you can afford to be a little more aggressive in picking an opener. You need to factor in how much the six prior lifts may have taken out of you, but you should select a weight that you can pull 10 times out of 10.

Remember, you are only selecting your *opening attempts.* You can change them (up or down) if you go to the scorer's table before your flight begins lifting.

My strategy for a lifter over age 50 is to treat your nine attempts as if the opener was your last warm up weight, and the next two were what you put 95% of your energy into. You will be amazed how much full power lifts will take out of you in a contest, so I recommend using a strategy that focuses most of your energy on the second and third attempts.

One additional thing you need to do to complete the registration for the meet. You need to get the "rack height" for your squat and bench press. All modern meets have adjustable height squat racks and bench press racks. You will have an opportunity to go on the platform and try different rack heights so that the loaders will have the bar in perfect position for you when you walk on the platform for your attempt.

You record your rack height on the meet registration/score card and give it to the official at the scorer's table. Now you are ready to compete when your flight is called.

Just before lifting begins for the day, one of the referees will call all the lifters together and give a briefing on the rules. You should know the rules before you get to the lifting venue, and have been practicing your lifts as if you were in a contest.

I have seen a lot of novice lifters blow some good lifts because they did not know the rules of performance. Know the rules of the federation you are lifting in. They can be found on line.

The Competition

Warming Up – In the section of this book called "practice everything" I suggest you adopt a warm up strategy that gets you ready to do your first attempt after doing only *four warm up reps.*

This is a trick taken straight from the martial arts where they have to train their bodies to go "from zero to sixty" almost instantaneously.

You can't do this if you have not practiced it. So, I suggest that you begin every training session warm up by working on doing absolute minimal warm up reps.

When you do this, you will find that you are totally ready to put out maximum effort after a few well selected reps. After I started doing this, I always enjoyed watching my competition begin by doing "ten reps with 135" and then sets of 5, 3, 3, and 1. All of the unnecessary expenditure of energy detracted from the juice they could put into their competition attempts.

How much energy will you save? As a rule of thumb, I always felt that a conservative warm up could be worth anywhere from 10-30 pounds in the squat, 10-20 in the bench press and up to 40 in the deadlift. You may not see all of those numbers every meet, but over time you will notice a positive difference.

Remember, you are there to win the contest…not the workout.

Here is an example of my minimal warm up sets (at age 72 weighing 180 lbs):

Squat: 135 x 2, 225 x 1, 275 x 1 – open at 325

Bench: 135 x 1, 185 x 1, 225 x 1 – open at 250

Deadlift: 135 x 1, 225 x 1, 315 x 1 – open at 375

You need to work into this type of warm up over time so your body gets used to it. Again, all reps with perfect form.

The Squat: your flight is now on the platform!

Assume for the moment that you are in the first flight of the day, and you have finished your warm ups. Now it is ShowTime!

You will be sitting in an area near the lifting platform called the "on deck area". All the other lifters in your flight will be there, along with some of their coaches and people helping them get ready to go on the platform when their name is called.

The announcer will begin by calling the names of the first five people in the lifting order. Assume for the moment that you are number 7 out of 12 in the flight on the first attempt.

The announcer will regularly call the next five lifters in the order they will go on the platform. The order will change as people lift, and your turn comes closer and closer. Eventually, you will be the lifter "on deck". That means you are the next one to lift.

What happens now will become familiar, but may be a blur at first. When the lifter ahead of you finishes their attempt, the scorer will tell the loaders what weight to put on the bar for you. It may take them a few moments to get the exact weight put on the bar, and the collars tightened.

At this point, you should be putting chalk on your hands. Chalking your hands for squatting will insure that your hands wont slip at any point during the lift. Chalking also gives some of us a small mental prompt. Chalk on the hands means it is Show Time!

At that point, the head referee will call "bar is loaded". Once this is called, _you have one minute_ to begin your lift. You should be ready to go on the platform the instant the head ref makes this call.

If you don't get the bar on your back and begin your descent within the one-minute time limit, you will forfeit the attempt. The loaders will load weight on the bar for the next lifter.

The spotters and loaders will have the squat bar set on the competition squat rack at the height you specified during check in. You walk up to the bar and set your hands in place first, then position the bar on your back the way you should have done in practice many many times.

There will be between three and five spotters on the platform with you. One will be behind you and the others will be at the end of the bar. They are there to help you if you lose control of the lift. They cannot touch you or the bar if you are going to have a legal lift.

When your feet are positioned properly, stand up with the bar and insure that it is balanced on your back. If something is not the way you want it, put the bar back on the rack and set up again. When the bar is steady across your shoulders, step back to the place where you will do your squat attempt.

You should have been practicing getting your feet in position to squat with no more than four steps. See the instructions in the chapter on squatting about doing a quick set up for squatting. You only need to step back far enough to clear the squat rack, not walk halfway across the platform.

You will see several lifters who take a lot of steps to get in position. All the while the bar is crushing down on them. This takes a great deal out of them. I always loved to see my opponents take seven to ten steps to get in position.

Remember, the clock is running while you do this. Assume that if you have practiced the set up and walk out, you will probably have nearly 30-40 seconds remaining on the clock when you are ready for the referee's command to squat.

Now you are positioned to begin your squat. You should nod your head to the head referee, and wait for the command to "squat". Once you begin to descend in the squat, the time clock goes off.

Once the head referee says "squat", you descend and do a complete squat, then return to exactly the same position you were in when the ref told you to squat. Your knees should be straight and your body upright. Stand there with the bar on your back and don't move...until the referee says "rack it".

If you put the bar back on the rack, or take a step toward the rack before you get the command from the referee, then you have "no lift". In other words, you have a big zero for all your effort, even if you did a perfect squat.

I'll say this over and over again...you _must know the rules._ You must practice your training lifts as if you were in a contest. Every lifting federation has their rules available on line. Know them cold...or you are likely to make a mistake that will cost you a lift.

Now...assume the ref has told you to "rack it". You take a step forward toward the squat rack and the spotters will help you get the bar back on the rack.

Let's also assume your lift was good. You will see the three referee's signals, usually a white or red paddle, or more likely lights illuminated on a large box that can be seen by everyone in the venue.

If one of the refs gives you a red light, this is the time to ask what you did wrong. A polite question will give you a quick answer.

Leave the lifting platform immediately. You now have _one minute_ to inform the scorer's table of your next attempt.

You should have made a plan before the meet on how much you wanted to increase the weight for your second attempt. Now, as you head to the scorer's table, you need to decide if your pre-contest plan is still the one you want to use.

Assuming you make you opening attempt, your body and intuition will tell you how big a jump to make for your second attempt. I found when I felt good, my second attempts tended to be close to the weight I did a single with at the end of my training cycle. When I didn't feel too good, I was more conservative.

The key thing is selecting a weight that you can do for a good lift. Picking a high weight that you miss gives you nothing on your total. If you make your second attempt, you can get very aggressive on your third attempt.

I can recall one meet in particular where the heat in the warm up area was so intense that all of us were getting cooked. Those of us who made allowance for this by lowering our attempts managed to get in three good lifts. They were lower than planned, but were successful. Lifters who ignored the heat wound up missing second and third attempts.

In short, listen to your body and pick a weight you can lift successfully.

Now another bit of advice. If you miss a lift, you should immediately ask the judges why you did not get a good lift. They will tell you quickly what they saw. It is important that you do this right away as most of us who have been in the referees' chairs will see hundreds of attempts on a given day, and it is hard to recall the details of a lift done hours or even minutes ago.

You should remember that referees in any major lifting federation will be experienced lifters themselves. They will also have been tested on the rules, and most have been required to do judging alongside a very experienced referee before they are certified to officiate. Many have been refereeing for years.

The point of this is that they are going to see things that casual observers and poorly shot videos are going to miss. Over the 22 years I spent as a referee, I can recall some occasions where lifters in their first meet insisted that they had done a perfect lift, when all three referees thought the opposite.

Recently, I have had people try to show me "video replays" of lifts that were called bad by three referees. In one case the three refs were multiple time world champions and had a combined refereeing experience of over 40 years. All three said "no lift", but the lifter was convinced that the phone video his buddy shot from a poor angle should be used to overturn the call.

The big problem with videos is pretty simple. Most are shot at an angle where you cannot accurately see depth on a squat, minor foot or hand movements, and in some cases whether the lifter complied with the referees calls to "start" or "rack".

If all three referees find a problem with a lift, there *was* a significant problem with the lift. The same applies if two out of three find a problem with the lift. In this case, you better find out what the problem IS so that you can correct it ASAP.

In the event you can't come up with a heavy squat, call for help from the spotters and they will quickly stabilize the weight and then help you stand erect and then get the bar back on the squat rack. Always stay with the bar. You and the spotters will get it back on the rack together.

Never EVER "dump" the bar backward. This is extremely dangerous to the spotters, especially the one standing behind you. It is also something that will get you thrown out of the meet. "Dump" a squat bar and your day of lifting is over right then.

Handling big iron is inherently dangerous. It can be downright scary for the spotters when someone is doing a big squat. I vividly recall being one of two end spotters on one end of a 900 lb squat attempt. Even with five spotters, 900 pounds is scary when you consider that the lifter could lose control and we would have to save him. The good news…the lift was successful.

For a lifter doing something as thoughtless and stupid as throwing a heavy barbell at the spotter behind you ranks at the top of the brainless scale. I talked about the practice of dumping weights that seems to be in vogue in Cross Fit. Suffice to say, this is extremely dangerous to the lifter and potentially crippling to the spotter.

By the time your third attempt comes in the squat, you will have survived your initial baptism of competitive lifting. If you have two good lifts in the books, you can be pretty aggressive on your third attempt. However, you really need to think about picking a lift you can actually do.

In general, lifters will be able to squat weights that are a bit lighter than they do in the gym. Being in a meet adds a considerable amount of tension and uncertainty that you don't face in the gym. You need to gage how much you can *actually* lift in front of the three referees you have and the crowd on hand.

Over the years I have heard all kinds of thoughts on selecting weights to lift from people who have never done a single lift in competition, or perhaps never competed in any organized sport. One of the most brain dead suggestions I have heard over and over is that "being in a meet will give you extra adrenalin, so you should be able to lift more in a meet than in the gym". Like I said…they have never been there and have no clue what they are talking about.

Don't fall for the thoughts of idiots who have never done a real competitive lift in front of referees. Competition is a whole different world than doing workouts.

With your squats completed, you now move to the bench press.

Bench Press

You will be warming up while another flight does their lifts. As a rule of thumb, I always estimate the time a flight will take to complete all three lifts as one minute per lift. For example, if there are 12 lifters in the flight, each will have three attempts so that is 3 x 12 which equals 36 minutes.

This is a rough estimate, and if the people loading the weights are capable and fast, the flight may go more rapidly.

In any event, you will be using a very few warm ups to get you ready to do your bench presses, so literally you can wait until the flight ahead of you is almost done before doing your warm ups.

There will also be some time needed to change the equipment on the platform from the squat to the bench press. This usually takes about five minutes unless the announcer tells you otherwise.

During the break between your squats and your bench press, I believe it is important to keep warm, and to insure you hydrate. Drink plenty of water during the meet. You would be amazed at how much water you will lose while competing.

You may want to eat something between lifts. This will depend on your own preference. However, I would strongly suggest that if you are going to eat something, it be small in size and easily digested. The last thing you want is to have a gut full of food when you are straining against your lifting belt pulling a deadlift.

Most meet directors insure that there is bottled water available for purchase, and occasionally for free. They may also have sports drinks like Gatorade. If you have planned ahead, you should have your own stash of food and drink in your equipment bag.

My own favorite story about staying hydrated came at the North American Championship meet in the tropical island of Aruba. I was lifting in support gear and the gym where the meet was being held was designed to be cooled by the normal tropical breezes. The breeze decided not to blow during the time I was lifting and the gym was like being in a sauna.

During the course of doing my three lifts, I downed three large bottles of Gatorade and two bottles of water. Over the course of the two and a half hours it took for our flight to complete their lifts, I lost 6 pounds! My body would have been trashed without all that hydration.

But now...on to the bench press.

You can change your opening attempt (the one you wrote on the registration/score card and gave to the scorer), if you want to. The rule is generally that you can change an opening attempt up to the time that the announcer calls your flight to begin lifting. If you are going to change your opener, do it as soon as you are clear that you want to do it.

My advice on selecting lifts in the bench press is much the same as I gave in the squat. Secure opener, increase for the second attempt based on how you feel on the first attempt, and the same logic for the third attempt.

Remember, you have to get at least one successful bench press in to be in the contest.

Some comments on the difference between competitive bench pressing and "gym" bench pressing.

First of all, you have to do the lift according to a referees' commands. If you don't wait for the command, your lift will not count. Second, the rules are very strict about pausing the weight on your chest before pushing upward. "Touch and go" lifts don't count. Third, when you are pressing the bar upward, any downward movement of the bar, even a tenth of an inch, means the lift does not count.

If those were not enough, you can't move your feet, your butt has to stay on the bench during the entire lift, and you have to wait for the command to "rack it" before putting the bar on the rack after you push it up.

Know the rules and practice your lifts in the gym as if you were in a meet. Do that and your responses in a meet will be automatic. If you don't practice your lifts according to the rules you will have to "think" about them all the time you are trying to put out full power. You will be wondering whether you are doing things right, rather than concentrating on the push.

But...back to the bench press.

The pace of the flight will be faster than the squat as the bench press is easier for the loaders to get the bar ready to lift. If the loaders are good, the total time each lifter uses for their attempt will be 30-40 seconds. That means that if you are in a flight of 12 lifters you will be making an attempt about every 8-9 minutes.

You will have a spotter standing at the middle of the bar right behind your head. Depending on meet rules, your coach can hand you the bar, or one of the spotters working at the meet. You can count on this person knowing what he is doing, and can arrange a simple hand off signal for when you want him to hand you the bar. (ex; "on three...").

There will also be at least one spotter on each end of the bar. They will have been trained by the meet director, so you can be confident that they will know what to do in the event you can't make the lift.

You should have been following the lifting order so that you are ready to walk on the platform as soon as the announcer calls your name. Chalk your hands...always. Wait at the side of the platform until the head referee calls out "bar loaded". Don't go on earlier, the loaders will be preparing the bar for your lift.

Once the referee calls "bar loaded", you have 60 seconds to get on the bench, take the hand off, get the referee's call to "start" and begin lowering the weight.

Likewise, you have one minute to inform the scorer's table of your next attempt.

Let's assume you have completed your bench press successfully, and will move on to the deadlift.

Deadlift: The money lift

There is a saying in golf that "you drive for show, and putt for dough". In other words, the money is made by the cats who are good at putting. The money lift in a powerlifting meet is the deadlift. It comes at the end of the contest, and is the lift that can very often wins the meet.

Because lifters can generally pull more weight in the deadlift than any other lift, it is possible to make up a significant deficit that a lifter might be in after the squat and bench press. Remember, it is the total of the three best lifts that wins.

Warm up carefully as described above, and be ready to go when your name is called to lift. Because the deadlift is technically easier than either the squat or bench press, you can be a little more aggressive in selecting your first lift.

At this point, you should know that I'm going to tell you to put chalk on your hands. This is worth at least 150-200 pounds of grip strength.

Most meets will have baby powder available to put on your thighs. This is to help the bar slide up your legs during the lock-out. In my opinion, baby powder is really good for making a mess, and marginally useful for lifting. If you get some on your hands, you are kind of screwed since it will make your hands slippery...not what you want.

Remember, get one solid lift to keep you in the meet, and then go after your competitors.

Because the deadlift is comparatively straightforward to do, it is not the time to get sloppy about your technique. I recall pulling a lift one time that was surprisingly light and as a result I moved one foot. Rules violation - No lift!

Like all the other lifts, you must *know the rules*. If you are going to do all the work of pulling the bar up, you need to know what is legal and what is not.

The biggest difference in selecting weights for the deadlift from all the lifts before is that on the last attempt, you have to put in your desired weight one minute after leaving the platform after your second attempt...BUT (and this is big), you can *change* your attempt once you see how the lifter immediately ahead of you does with their attempt.

I used this at the IPF Masters World Championships in Pretoria, South Africa in 2005 to win the silver medal instead of taking bronze. The lifter immediately ahead of me failed in their attempt, so I could go for the silver. My coach submitted the weight to the scorer immediately on seeing the lifter ahead of me fail on his pull, and I was able to successfully pull my weight to win the silver.

I'll assume you have a solid pull on the first two lifts and are wondering what you might try on the third attempt. If your body says "I'm up for a personal record attempt", then go for it. If your bod says "I'm done for today", then honor that. You will be utterly amazed at how much energy you have expended over the two to three hours you have been lifting.

The last activity of the day will be the awards ceremony. At that time you will get an award for being in the event. At this point I hope you will be feeling a sense of satisfaction. Powerlifting is for lions and tigers…not the meek.

Remember the words of Teddy Roosevelt:

> "It is not the critic who counts; not the man who points out how the strong man stumbles, or where the doer of deeds could have done them better. The credit belongs to the man who is actually in the arena; who's face is marred by dust and sweat and blood; who strives valiantly; who errs, who comes up short again and again, because there is no effort without error and shortcoming; but who does actually strive to do the deeds; who knows the great enthusiasms, the great devotions; who spends himself in a worthy cause; who at the best knows in the end the triumph of high achievement, and who at the worst, if he fails while daring greatly, so that his place shall never be with those cold and timid souls who know neither victory nor defeat…."

After Action Review: What did I learn?

To keep improving, it is essential that you learn something from every meet. What went right and why, what was a problem, and what were some new and different things you saw that could be of benefit next time?

Sitting down right after a meet and making a detailed assessment of things you want to do better, things you want to do the same, and things you want to investigate will really help you keep getting better.

I always learned something from every meet in which I competed, from every meet where I refereed, and from every meet I put on as a meet director. You can always learn something new and valuable.

It will usually be little things that taken together can make a big difference. But, getting them written down when they are fresh in your mind is very important. A few days later, you may have forgotten something important.

If you have a coach, it will help if you do this with him or her. How can you work better as a team? What does the coach think you need to work on as opposed to what you think you need? Being systematic and comparing notes will be of great benefit for your continuing improvement.

Afterword

I look back on 60 years of training and competing in a variety of different sports my main feeling is one of gratitude. I have had the opportunity to participate in many sports, meet a lot of very different people and reap the benefits of having great health.

Long ago I learned that it is impossible to achieve anything significant if you don't love the process of training and preparation. In my professional life I often had the feeling that I was really lucky that I got paid me to do something I would have done for free because I enjoyed it so much.

So it is with power training. I have never met anyone who competed who didn't completely enjoy the process of "getting there".

It is my sincere hope that you find the joy and sense of being completely alive that comes when you "lift heavy stuff" for a few hours a week.

Enjoy the journey.

Made in the USA
Middletown, DE
04 June 2025

76530521R00166